HEALTH, HEALING
&
HAPPINESS

Mary-Joy Payten

HEALTH, HEALING & HAPPINESS

Copyright © Mary-Joy Payten

First published 2023

ISBN: 978-0-6457342-5-6 Paperback

ISBN: 978-0-6457342-6-3 E-Book

Cover Design by Mary-Joy Payten.

Graphics by Rod Lane.

Photograph of author by Luke Feltham.

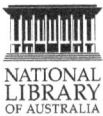

NATIONAL LIBRARY OF AUSTRALIA

A catalogue record for this book is available from the National Library of Australia

Disclaimer: The information contained in this book is for educational purposes only; it should not be used for diagnosis or to guide treatment without the opinion of a health professional. Any reader who is concerned about his or her health should contact a licensed medical professional.

Contents

A

B

C

D

E

F

G

H

I

N

O

P

Q

R

S

T

U

V

FOREWORD

Dear Reader

I wouldn't be here today if it wasn't for our house burning to the ground in Springwood, in the Blue Mountains (west of Sydney). This happened when I was 5 years old during the Second World War and my father was a padre in New Guinea. We lost everything except for a sewing machine in a wooden cabinet. I still remember standing across the street watching and what my nightie looked like.

The firemen had been aiming at the beautiful round Lazy Susan type fridge (few people owned fridges at that time) with the neighbour's food rations inside it, as it was so much better than an ice-block cooler. The recently oiled sewing-machine cabinet (after making new clothes for my father's arrival home) was beside it. I still remember standing in my nightdress, watching the house burn down from across the road.

My mother, 2 younger sisters and I had to go to a boarding house the day after the fire wearing clothes from boys across the road, much to my horror. Girls didn't usually wear jeans and T-shirts in those days, only dresses.

The owner of the boarding house took one look at me and told my mother to take me to Sydney to see Bernard Jansen, who was a masseur, naturopath, iridologist, herbalist, homeopath, astrologer (I'm a Libra) and theosophist. Only found out about the last 2 in my adult years.

Sadly, the fridge went but not the sewing machine. It looked like a burned log for many years until it was finally painted over.

When my father come home (I didn't recognise him) and we moved to Sydney, the sewing machine was used endlessly for years to come. We saved money by making and altering clothes in the poor suburb (at that time) of Clovelly. My father, as a minister, believed that God would provide.

We were literally as poor as church mice, wearing the second-hand clothing donated to charity and often redesigned. Thank God for the old sewing machine. The situation was so bad that my mother, on the quiet, scrubbed floors for some parishioners. Thankfully, some years later members of the church ran a big fundraiser to enable the Reverend to have a car. It was life changing in many ways.

At the time of the fire, I was dying of a heart problem (murmur), and in those days doctors said there was nothing they could do about it. I would just slow down and die.

I heard this story many times as a child and became very fearful at the slightest pain that I was dying. Often stayed awake sitting at the window looking out over the view, thinking that it might be my last night. It wasn't until I was 18, when a psychic told me I would live a long life, that I lost some of the fear. However, it still springs up sometimes when I have an unknown pain in my chest-and-throat area. More recently, psychics say I could live to be very old. I'm now 82.

As a child, I used to have dizzy turns and fall (landed on a bee once and got stung), once when being minded at school while Mother shopped with my sister in the stroller. We lived a mile or so from the shops with no transport, and I still remember those miserable walks in hot, windy summer. I suffered a terrible body cramp up to my heart. I wanted to scream but didn't as the teacher was doing my mother a favour. In my early years I became a stoic, as my mother called it. Just like my father. In some ways I took his place; hence unlikely to complain about anything.

The other problem I had was a turned left eye. My parents couldn't afford the operation on my eye, so there was lots of exercise instead, which I hated. I wore a patch for years over the other eye to make the weak eye work.

These health issues started when I was 2 years old, after I went to hospital – a perfectly healthy child with a bad case of measles. From recent reading, I now know that I would have caught a virus in hospital and more than likely still have it.

Luckily my mother was open minded enough to go to Mr Jansen once we moved to Sydney. She had also sent a letter seeking healing from a famous healer in the UK. As I improved, although the massage was extremely painful and the herbal medicine ghastly, my mother used to say, "Our fire was God given". Otherwise, I would have died. By the time I was 12, I had a clean bill of health, including a straight eye.

In my Forties, I spent a lot of time healing emotionally and developing self-esteem. I learned to stop being a people pleaser and how to really communicate. Still learning.

For over 75 years, all the things I experienced and learned, including all the emails with health hints, mean that my family and I have used natural methods to look after our health when possible, and I want to share this knowledge with you.

When you have a health problem start with do-it-yourself info, Naturally go to the doctor if not getting results. I do believe in some of the wonders of modern medicine and the great effort and work that many doctors do.

A good natural therapist and counsellor will always advise you to go to the doctor if they think it is the only way to heal whatever is wrong. Natural therapies can be complementary with medication. Many doctors today study both Western medicine and one or two of the natural therapies as well. This is especially true in several European countries, particularly in Germany.

I believe in preventative medicine, which is what Chinese medicine is about. People visit their doctor regularly to stay healthy rather than wait until they have a disease. All forms of healing are complementary. I do annual check-ups with iridology and live blood even if I feel OK. Some things show up as developing or in need of balancing, so early treatment prevents the problem reaching the symptom level.

HOW TO READ THIS BOOK

I want to talk and share with you what I think, know and feel at times. Therefore, it is not scientific, though sometimes autobiographical. Mainly it comprises comments regarding my and others' experiences and what I think about some subjects.

There is a list of all kinds of subjects in alphabetical order. The subjects cover herbs, environment, emotions, vegetables, fruit, meat, seafood, chemical, electromagnetic fields and all types of causes and healing methods. There are references to acupuncture, astrology, naturopathy, osteopathy, herbalism, reflexology, Reiki, Iridology and emotional issues that I believe, and know from experience, can have considerable effects on my health.

Today, many doctors and scientists are aware of the emotional and lifestyle issues that can create poor health and are advising people to take these into account when showing symptoms.

I know some of the methods and herbs will not be to your taste or will seem too hard to do. I have certainly experienced this and am quite surprised that following some of the suggestions, even from personal experience, other people won't do them because of the taste or pain. **What is more important than getting well – taste or healing/preventing diseases?** Increasingly we want instant gratification, which is why pills (drugs) are so popular to fix everything, though the pills have side effects and the problem often returns. Complementary healing can be slower, though not always.

Drugs are now becoming a worry as they have been over prescribed and people don't finish what they are taking if feeling okay (I've done it too). The worst thing is it gets into the water supply when thrown out or via their urine.

Now they are worried about superbugs and what our own bodies are becoming immune to as the prescriptions once appeared to heal, though they often don't get to the cause and the problem can re appear. This is happening to people after they have their Covid 19 jab.

Originally, drugs were made from natural ingredients. Vaccination is a part of this. Homeopathy is very much like vaccination, as it is about giving a small amount of the problem to develop immunity. Unfortunately, vaccinations now are made from a lot of ingredients that can have a very bad effect on a person, such as aluminium and mercury. In the past they could be given at a time or in an amount that a doctor thought suitable for a child (as they are all different) but not now.

The hard thing to face is that usually it has taken a long time for us to reach this point of illness because of constant stress, poor eating and health habits. The body has managed to work okay but has finally given up and shown that it can't continue to support you.

I've heard people when getting an eye diagnosis (Iridology) say, "Why should I give up this or that – I'm fine". The Iridologist will say, "That may be true but it is showing a weakness now, and if you don't change a few habits you will have a health problem in that area in the future".

Sometime later they return, maybe years later, needing a cure for something they had been warned about long ago. This certainly happened in my family several times. I know changing the food and medicine is hard, and this also applies to setting a routine, but worth it.

So, I say be brave, do it, eat it, drink it and think of how much good it is doing you. Whatever you eat, good or bad, say "Everything I eat makes me happy and healthy".

There are several books available regarding the all-round causes of disease – mental, emotional, physical, spiritual and metaphysical – which include affirmations for health.

When talking with friends they often ask for suggestions regarding their health. They wonder about certain things like their star signs, things they are eating, etc. and ask is it "good or bad".

I always say, "Most things are neither good nor bad; they just are". Too much or too little of anything can be good or bad for you. It is what you do with it that makes it good or bad.

The first thing to is do when you get a pain or health problem is check my Louise Hay's book as to the metaphysical cause and take note of the affirmation. You could do some massage in the area if it is easy to reach. Then think about whether you need to go to a healer and which type of healing would be best.

You can also look at the Astrology section in this book as to what part of the body is being affected by your emotions and colours you might use or avoid in food and what you wear. All check the Cell Salts out to see if there is something there that can help like for cramp.

I do know that resolving health issues, when due to imbalance (dis-ease) is related to our emotional, mental, physical and spiritual state brings healing and happiness.

There are other books within the context of the subject, but these ones I found so enlightening that they may answer your questions:

Heal your body: The mental causes for physical illness and the metaphysical way to overcome them by Louise Hay. Hay has written many more books, but I find this so simple and easy to understand. When people say they have a certain symptom, I check my *Little blue book* (family name for it) and people will say "Yes, that's how I feel". What I like is that it includes the backbone and all the problems one can have if the back is not aligned.

The secret language of your body: The essential guide to health and wellness by Inna Segal. This is a terrific book written from a self-healing perspective and includes colours as well as emotional causes.

Love your disease It's keeping you healthy: by John Harrison. This is a real eye opener to the unconscious feelings creating disease, e.g. asthma developing at a late age.

The body keeps the score: Mind, brain and body in the transformation of trauma by Bessel van der Kolk. The author discusses changing the tracks to the brain caused by action and thoughts, as well as traumatisation from early childhood.

Edgar Cayce, born 18 March 1877 and died in 1945, was known as the **"Sleeping Prophet"** and had many books printed based on his readings and the amazing healings he achieved with thousands of people.

Cayce became famous mainly through his readings of clients covering past lives and by discovering the source of the illness and how to cure it even using Coca-Cola (Coke), which amazed me when nothing else had worked.

There is an Edgar Cayce Foundation continuing his work in Virginia USA and branches around the world, including Australia.

I wish you all the luck, courage, support, energy, will and whatever it takes to supplement and complement your medicines and add to and improve your everyday food and lifestyle, knowing it brings you **HEALTH, HEALING & HAPPINESS.**

INTRODUCTION

Healing is through medical, physical, mental, emotion, spiritual and lots of patience. This is an example I am using. It addresses my current experience using this form of healing with LOVE.

AGED MACULAR DEGENERATION (AMG) – They say no cure for dry; only wet.

My situation suddenly appeared October '21 though I had my eyes checked about 6 months before. Somehow, I wasn't happy with the blurring when reading and things were beginning to have strange shapes. I had no idea that they were symptoms of AMG. Thought it started with a black hole in my vision first.

Went to the optometrist and she was surprised I had developed cataracts in such a short time so sent me to the specialist. He wasn't worried about those but said I had wet AMG.

The cure was to have an initial jab in the eye once a month for 3 months then space them out, depending on how well it is working, to stop the growth. I think it was caused by me spending many more hours on the internet than usual due to writing a book and masses of emails re Covid etc: less outside in the fresh air and sun, plus stress.

Also, I looked at the metaphysical reasons related to childhood eye problems and what I needed to look at in my life now that could be related to the current situation.

I held off the jab for a month as it sounded dreadful to jab my eye. Told the doctor that I wanted to see what my natural therapists said. (Someone I know has had 40 jabs over the years.) Meanwhile, my darling sister hunted the internet and had lots of suggestions.

At the beginning, everyone said I needed the needle as there was no cure. The natural therapy articles said it may well be improved by approaching it from many angles, such as certain foods and cutting down stress.

It was getting worse, so I went for the jab to stop further deterioration. However, from the time of diagnosis, I had started taking some herbal mixture which I got from the naturopath that might help. The specialist knew of it but said it wouldn't cure, which of course it wouldn't on its own, and not quickly.

As well as doing the things below, I had a test at the third-monthly needle and I was quite improved as the fluid had gone. Next time I went after 6 weeks, and it hadn't gotten any worse (I had been having fairly clear vision by then). So, he said make it 3 months next time as it has been okay until now, April. Though once it was 4 months and okay.

Recently I said I want to leave it longer as I have had no symptoms for a year and it is very expensive. He said the makers of the medicine say every 3 months so he follows that. How come it isn't up to the doctor to decide? Finally, he said it was my choice and he said 4 months. I told him it would be my responsibility. Obviously, they don't think it can be cured or don't leave it long enough to find out. I will keep extending it from now on and see what happens. Will tell the doctor then that I intend to go 5 months and so on. If people are told they will never walk and do, why can't my eye heal? Have to cross that bridge when I come to it.

After the first 4 months, I had felt ready to get some new glasses as I'd been juggling glasses for reading and broken ones. The optometrist informed me that my eyesight was better than before I was diagnosed.

Maybe not all of this is important or you would want to do them, but this is a list of things I have done:

Most pills are taken once a day, so I put half in the cupboard with breakfast things and the other half separately to take at night. If twice a day, I move them backward and forward.

Affirmation and visualising: "I have clear vision" and I am grateful for healing and for the healers whenever I think about it. Also, I use **colour affirmations and clearing** from the book **The Secret Language of Your Body** by Inna Segal.

Blue-light glasses: they block the blue rays from the computer entering the eye. Got some for $10 at Aldi, which broke. Later found some at Chemist Warehouse. Check the internet. I put them on over my normal glasses. Some people have it incorporated in their glasses, but I don't think that is good for ordinary daily vision.

Eye bath: once or twice a day with filtered water. Sometimes add mineral salt and I sometimes do drops of colloidal silver into my eye as it is a bacteria killer. During bathe time I roll my eyes in different directions – side, back, circular – and do each session until they stop stinging. Then they are clean.

Exercise and Meditation: I walk most mornings along the Broadwater, Gold Coast. A good time to energise and use affirmations. I find meditation difficult; my mind races, but this is a form of meditation.

However, if windy or bad weather, I can use a video I have which is isometric and from the '90s or I make an L-shape yoga position with bum against the wall and legs up the wall for 10 minutes. Then I use my Zen-chi machine lying on the floor shaking all over, which goes for 15 minutes. All good for circulation.

Reiki: hands on self when possible.

Sunshine: as the eyes take a good deal of our energy each day, they build up toxins. The way to clear them, apart from bathing, is to be in the sun without sunglasses. I close my eyes and face the sun for about 5 to 10 minutes to cleanse the toxins. Reading in the sun wearing a hat with no glasses improves the eyesight too.

Sunglasses: they block the eyes from absorbing the vitamins and healing, though others say it keeps you safe from cancer. Follow what you feel is right. Like most things, do it in moderation.

Years ago, I couldn't do without sunglasses but found wearing a brim hat or visor cut the glare, and driving with the sun visor down does the job (wish the car visors had ones that short people can use successfully when the sun is low). Between 10 and 4 is the best time to avoid the sun except being out in it for 20 minutes to absorb vitamin D which is only in that time span. Of course sunnies are good if skiing or beaching for any length of time.

Foods and Herbs

Any dark-blue berries, **yellow** vegies, carrot and fruit are also good for the vitamin A. Pawpaw, papaya and pineapple are real antioxidants with very high potential of hydrogen (pH) factor for healing.

Astaxanthin 12 mg: supports skin structure, clears free radicals, and much more.

Goji berries are also good for the eyes. I often have them in my porridge.

Herbal mix: ginkgo 50 ml and bilberry 60 ml. Take 3 ml once **a day in a little water..**

Orthoplex: Eye Rite extra strong vitamin A for eyes.

Performance lab: Vision (from UK) eye pills. Take one once a day. Some herbs mentioned below are in this product and it is okay to take as well as the pills because they aren't strong enough to clash. In fact, I am now not continuing with them as I prefer to take the main products rather than a mild mix.

Vitamin A is essential for skin and eyesight.

Zeaxanthin: kiwi fruit is high in this. You can buy pills separately though again it is in the Vision pills but I've just upped my kiwi fruit.

I am now easing off some of the pills and herbal mix suggested above as I don't think it is urgent now. Must keep with vitamin A though and the fruit and vegetables.

Further suggestions

Saffron: 20 mg a day is good but I haven't yet followed up. There is a farm where they make this on the Sunshine Coast and sell ointments and other products at markets. On the net, people were saying their eyes had improved using the product.

Cod-liver oil: I haven't used it for a few years but have started again as it's good for my joints, which are clicking a bit, and omega 3. The one I got has "Vision" written on the label under "cod-liver oil".

Naturally, I regularly take zinc, vitamin C and vitamin D in the morning and magnesium at night. Before bed I take a few cell salts like magnesium phosphate (mag phos for short) to relax muscles and silica to cleanse.

One of my healers tells me that a lot of his patients are using **hemp oil** and it is doing a lot for their eyes. His patients say the optometrists are surprised at improvement. Start with 1 teaspoon and go to 4 teaspoons a day. It is also very good for many other health problems. Similar situation I think with **cannabis oil.**

A

ACHES and PAINS

We often have strange aches and pains and can start to worry about them if they are around for more than a day or two.

I say "Thank God" for having done Reiki 1 and 2 back in the '80s. I put my hands on the sore spot and usually it clears. Also great for cold feet using the circulation area (the groin) learned in Reiki 1. I also massage myself in the area which is in pain. Often massaging until it clears – as a lot of pains are congestion of some kind in the area.

If pain continues for a longer time, I will often go to the osteopath (who includes massage **before** adjusting, which is what chiropractor does), or naturopath, or to acupuncturist, even reflexologist. Depends on the type of pain.

This has meant, much to my surprise, that the problem is somewhere else in the body. Many pains go back (via the meridian) to the source of the nerves in the spine that feed the blood and energy to the area.

Of course, if there is still no relief, go to the doctor.

ACUPUNCTURE

I've been amazed at what acupuncture can heal. It certainly can take pains away, often for conditions that the doctor can't find on answer to – for example my getting dizzy and not having energy or feeling too nauseous to do anything. One treatment and I am up and running. Tells me it is imbalance of ying and yang or stagnant chi.

A numb toe ends up being a problem with gall bladder. Two treatments – gone.

AFFIRMATION and THOUGHTS

There are many books on this subject, and after reading them you will be inspired to use them. It helps us question our thoughts and how we end up getting what we are thinking about. Thoughts create things.

Always start an affirmation with "I am ... I want ... I feel ...." and really feel what it is I want, imagine it, really believe it. Many people have a cut-out board on their desk or wall with a picture of what it is they want. You can have a few affirmations going at the same time. Write your wishes out and put them under your pillow round the new moon. Maybe even leave them there for a while.

Don't think about what you don't want, only about what you **do** want, as the universe will create it for you both good and bad. As they say, "Where the mind goes, the energy flows".

Every time you say "I have ...", you are affirming it, and that includes diseases, but it could be about love or money, etc. No poor thoughts about money. Say "It's not in my budget at the moment", not "I can't afford it". Avoid affirming your disease as much as possible. Say something like "I'm not well at the moment".

Using words like "Should" makes you feel guilty or you are blaming someone. When we say "Could" meaning "Can you ...", (of course you can), it means you may not be able to do something so simple as take the bin out. "Would" means a wish you have like "Would you take the bin out?" Try these words out and see how they make you feel.

Once I asked my mother for a beach towel for Christmas but not autumn colours. Surprised to get an autumn colour towel.

I sent an invitation out once asking people to wear pastel colours, no dark colours. I was shocked to see some people who often wear pastels turn up in dark colours.

The universe doesn't understand "No", "Not" or "Don't". It only picks up the words. Also, often people don't recognise them either when it comes to using them. Many people just keep on doing or saying what they want. So instead of saying, "Don't do that to me" (giving them the power), take your power back and say, "I won't be treated like that," and mean it in a very firm voice or "So what" putting it back to their responsibility. You can say nasty things to people in a sweet, soft voice, and they take no notice.

So, whatever you want changed, healed or improved on when you start to think about it, STOP and affirm what you want. I have a collection of about 4 affirmations about current issues that I use while walking and whenever I start worrying about an issue.

AIR CONDITIONING

The **car** manual says to roll down the windows to let out all the hot air before turning on the air conditioning. WHY? Can be another reason people are dying from cancer more than ever before.

Many people are in their cars the first thing in the morning and the last thing at night, 7 days a week. They turn on the air conditioner as soon as they get in the car. It is suggested that you open the windows after you get in and then, after a couple of minutes, turn on the air conditioning.

It seems that all the nooks and crannies, plastic, etc. emit benzene, which is a cancer-causing toxin. It also can cause anaemia and affect the bones, kidneys, reducing white blood cells. In a hot climate, these toxins will be very strong. Once absorbed into the body, it is very hard to expel, and we are mostly unaware of it until illness arrives.

Most people in a modern home have a door (which is often left open) into the house from the garage. When the garage door is down, all the toxins and bad air float into the house. This is even worse if the car is reversed with its back to the door. When it starts, the fumes project into the house.

In our **homes,** the air conditioning along with fans can circu-late toxins and poor-quality air. I find sitting under or in front of an air conditioner or fan can cause coughing, throat problems, a cold and headaches. I usually carry a shawl/pashmina when I go out (matching of course) in case I am in a draft from the fans and air con. Sometimes I must move seating or even leave.

I'm not sure for how long I didn't recognise the situation, certainly once living in the tropics or holidaying there, but it has got worse recently here in the subtropics. I find people put the air-con on hot or cool and overhead fans on full blast, winter and summer. Maybe having the fans on low speed will help, but people seem to forget that hot air rises and cold air sinks. I'm inclined to think they contradict each other, especially if the overhead fans are not adjusted.

AIR POLLUTION
– see Autism and many other conditions

It seems from research that young children exposed to toxic air pollutants are significantly more likely to develop autism as their brains are more vulnerable

Most people are affected by vehicle exhausts, road dust, emissions from factories and construction works. Pollutants from these sources can lead to lack of fertility, stroke, heart disease, lung cancer and shorter lives.

Some places are so chronic where people almost live in a fog, which must create shorter lives. Even when people know they should move, they cannot as they have nowhere to go or the necessary money to do so.

ALZHEIMER'S
– see B vitamins, Dementia, Coconut oil, Cannabis

I have read quite a bit regarding aluminium being found in the brains of people with this disease. Therefore, it is important to use stainless-steel saucepans, steel or enamelled. If non stick (now much safer than previously) don't use metal utensils as once scratched they are toxic

Alzheimer's and grey matter loss need vitamin B, carrots, green tea along with other foods such as green leafy vegetables, nuts, berries, fish and olive oil. Now, there are many things' people can do and take to avoid or improve the situation.

ANKLES
– see Acupuncture, Feet, Slapping

Ankles and lower legs often begin to have problems as we get older. This can take the form of ulcers, skin cancer, weakness, aching, etc. Doctors always say that poor circulation is one of the causes of lack of healing.

Something you can do is lie with bottom against a wall and put your legs up the wall. Doing this for up to 20 minutes is good for circulation. I have found that I get feeling in my throat, round my head sometimes almost immediately, and the blood is now being forced through my body.

Slapping the soles of your feet, round your ankles and legs is stimulating. Whenever watching television or reading, put your feet up on something like a stool or coffee table, rather than have them hang to the ground, this helps the circulation.

ANXIETY

I have found so much anxiety is often needless worry over something that may happen and quite often doesn't. Therefore, it is wasting time and energy and can cause pain, lack of sleep and sickness. Also worrying about other people's situations which I can do nothing about ruins my sleep.

So, it is much better to have a plan in case a situation doesn't happen and then stop thinking about it – mainly by changing the subject of your thoughts to something happy or more positive.

I know, I know it's very hard as I'm a born worrier, but it helps. What also helps if unable to sleep is to get up and write it out. Getting it off your chest seems to make a big difference. You'll find you can go back to sleep.

ARMS – see Hands

Pains down the arms can be for all sorts of reasons, but it is usually due to stress and tension in your neck, shoulders and further down your spine.

I get a lot of pain at times in my arms, only to find out from my acupuncture, massage man that it is stress in the muscles round the heart. We have meridians from our heads going down to our fingertips.

You can also massage your hands, fingers and palm until the pain eases or stops.

ASPARTAME

Aaspartame is carcinogenic.

There have been several tests on this, and scientists have found that it can cause a wide range of malignancies in rodents. Therefore, it would have a bad effect on people.

Recently, a test on men drinking a lot of diet soda, which contains aspartame, found they had a higher risk of non-Hodgkin's lymphoma and myeloma, compared to men who don't drink it.

The best sweetener to use is Stevia, (or honey) which is made from a plant. You can get it in powder or liquid, and the little one with drops for your tea or coffee easily fits into your pocket.

ASPIRIN

Most heart attacks occur in the day, generally between 6 am and noon.

Having one during the night, when the heart should be most at rest, means that something unusual happened. It seems sleep apnea is to blame.

People are now taking aspirin, which is a blood thinner, when going to bed so the body system can absorb it.

I have found if I go to bed with aches round my shoulder blades or arms, head feeling blocked, I take an aspirin sometimes and when I wake all is OK. This also applies to feeling like I'm going down with a cold. I have a lemon drink and take 2 aspirin. Usually, all okay in the morning. This is due to the fact they are also anti-inflammatory.

One evening I called the ambulance as I had pain round the left jaw, throat, arm and found it hard to breathe. I told them I took an Aspro, and they asked which one, and they said I had done the right thing and it was the right Aspro. I use the basic, original one, not all the other versions.

Many people are opposed to them as they say they have all sorts of side effects on the gut, but I find the occasional one works well.

ASTHMA

Many people have found that various breathing styles, acupuncture, massage and spinal adjustments can be of great help with this, along with understanding where the source could be emotionally and avoiding some foods.

A young gay man, who I worked with, suddenly got asthma. I asked him what he had been getting emotional about. He said the new boss was causing him a lot of stress, and I suggested he should learn to deal with the stress and recognise how upsetting it was to his health.

A few weeks later, he came up to me and said he had stopped having asthma. I was a bit shocked and asked him how. It seems that he had been at a party and forgot to bring his puffer, so he decided, "Damn it. I'm not going to let the boss get me down and ruin my health. Stuff him". Seemed to do the trick as it was so firm and believed.

Obviously, it can be much more complicated than that, but having read about it happening in a similar way in **Love your disease: It's keeping you healthy** by John Harrison, I know it can be done immediately.

ASTROLOGY AND HEALTH

Many people specialise in the health side of astrology, which is very complicated. Back before the age of science began, most doctors used astrology along with their herbal medicines.

Today we find that different astrology signs (also where their planets have moved to) and temperaments do well with using homeopathic treatments, cell salts and herbal treatments.

Some scientists label certain temperaments as more likely to get certain diseases and many astrologers can help with diagnoses. This includes mental and emotional situations.

One psychologist/counsellor I knew would do a chart for the person by getting their birthday when they made their appointment and found she could tune into the problem long before all the talking around the bush came up with the problem.

This is a list of possible effects related to the astrology sign and the colour associated:

Aries rules the head, face, sinuses, blood, and the muscular system: RED.

Taurus rules the neck, throat, and voice: GREEN.

Gemini rules the shoulders, arms, and hands as well as the lungs (breathing): YELLOW.

Cancer rules the belly, breasts, uterus, and digestion generally: WHITE/SILVER.

Leo rules the spine, chest, heart, the cardiac system: GOLD.

Virgo rules the intestines and abdomen as well as the process of absorbing nutrients, minerals and vitamins from food: BROWN/ DEEP GREEN.

Libra rules the kidneys, bladder, ovaries, and the endocrine system: PINK/BLUE.

Scorpio rules the bowels, genitals, and organs of elimination: BLOOD RED/MAROON.

Sagittarius rules the thighs, hips, and buttocks, plus the sciatic nerve: DARK BLUE/PLUM.

Capricorn rules the skin, teeth, hair, nails, and bones – the entire skeletal system: BLACK/DARK BROWN/CHARCOAL.

Aquarius rules the ankles, calves, nerve impulses and the circulatory system: ELECTRIC BLUE/PURPLE.

Pisces rules the feet, toes, and the immune and lymphatic systems.

Pisces are happiest when their feet are well taken care of: MAUVE/SEA GREEN.

ADHD – ASPERGER'S – AUTISM – RSD

Many very successful and world-renowned people are now known to be on the spectrum so no longer a need to hide their problem. Now they inspire people to check themselves.

I think most of us have heard and read a great deal about attention-deficit hyperactivity disorder (ADHD).

As more adults are now being tested (not just children) and talking about it, this means that it is not ignored. They were considered mentally unwell in the past. People with a diagnosis feel great relief to find out what has caused so much trouble in their lives.

Asperger's

Asperger's is now on the spectrum used to define the kind of problems people have, starting with ADHD.

They don't seem to have any understanding of other people's needs or emotions and much more.

Autism

Autism is becoming a huge problem for children in the Western world at least, and sometimes there are several afflicted children in the one family. I can only name the problem but have no answer.

Rejection sensitive dysphoria (RSD)

Rejection sensitive dysphoria is not yet in the *Diagnostic and Statistical Manual of Mental Disorders* (DSM-5). However, there are web pages by Aaron Ansuini (2019) on the condition, and they really rang a bell with me as it seems more complicated than ADHD.

Ansuini was hyper-emotional, super-sensitive, a drama queen, overreacting to comments, ruining relationships because of exploding over the slightest comment taken personally, and demonstrated other similar behaviours.

It is suggested that Cognitive Behaviour Therapy is a helpful way to handle this problem, as well as the medication.

There are a lot of toxins related to ADHD and autism, including aluminium on the brain. Also, most lack vitamin D, which is absorbed from the sun and is necessary for bone and muscle development, and much more.

Many mothers have been low in vitamin D, and children are kept out of the sun because of skin-cancer worries. This could be one of the reasons for the problem. Therefore, it is important that people get some exposure to the sun.

Many doctors and natural therapists have blamed our modern lifestyle such as electronic radiation, vaccinations, mobiles, hormones, as well as food. This has come about since the '70s with the huge growing situation regarding these problems. Personally, I think there must be a link.

During the early '70s, a young boy in our family was said to be hyperactive, and today this behaviour would be on the autism spectrum. I think it was emotional trauma from a marriage breakup, moving from another country and being very physical, along with the need to be really involved with what he was learning. School didn't interest him. They said he would grow out of it. Didn't really happen, and life has been a hard act.

I suppose autism existed in the past, but I'd not heard of it until about the '80s though I had moved and travelled overseas a lot. Obviously, its prevalence was not anything like it is now.

ARTHRITIS AND RHEUMATISM

– Colloidal minerals, acupuncture

As I understand it, this is a build-up of acid in the body, so it is suggested that a change in eating habits can be helpful. Also, though it may be painful, massage can break up the congestion. Acupuncture can also ease the pain.

I think a copper bracelet may help as it certainly stopped my rheumatism, which I understand is similar to arthritis.

There are many minerals and foods which can be helpful. Being such a broad subject, I suggest you look on the internet for the natural healing or relief of it to use with your medication.

AUTOIMMUNITY

– see Baking Soda

The Body Keeps the Score: Mind, Brain and Body in the Transformation of Trauma by Bessel van der Kolk.

Autoimmunity and metal implants, devices, and vaccine adjuvants by Amanda Just and Jack Kall.

The above book and paper provide very good information on the subject, along with others.

Autoimmune conditions are thought to be related to metals in the system. Some people can't wear watches and jewellery or implants. The condition also has a strong connection to post-traumatic stress.

B

BABY CONCEPTION

Naturopaths, herbalists, homeopaths have helped people take the right foods and natural herbs to stimulate the process of conception.

Osteopaths have cleared tension, nerves and circulation blocks from the spine through manipulation. Also, acupuncture has also been helpful.

Sometimes after having some therapy, women have cleared up emotional blockages and fears, enabling them to conceive. It is well known that once some people adopt a child, they end up having their own child. This happened to a friend of mine, and she ended up with only 13 months between them.

Baby conception – sperm problems

Abstaining from alcohol and drugs prior to conceiving a child has usually been considered the woman's responsibility. Now, at last, it is understood both parents need to reduce their intake of alcohol and poor food.

The main concern surrounding alcohol exposure during pregnancy often relates to well-established evidence of newborns developing a range of behavioural, physical and cognitive disabilities later in life.

Studies show that paternal alcohol consumption and poor diet have a negative effect at all levels of the male reproductive system. This is as well as altered neurological, behavioural and biochemical outcomes in subsequent generations.

I know of one couple who were having problems, and the doctor advised them that they would be more likely to conceive by stopping weed and any other drugs plus cutting the drinking right down. It took a few months, but they were thrilled to have conceived.

Imagine if all those kings, princes, etc. stopped blaming women for their lack of sons when the situation might well have been due to their own unhealthy lifestyles. The world would be a different place now.

BAKING SODA – BICARB

– see Cancer – PH – Flu

I suggest you visit the Mercola Video Library by Dr Mercola (American prices and products). There is a lot of information on all kinds of diseases, healing and diets.

I've known for some years that baking soda, or sodium bi-carbonate, which is in homes for baking and cleaning, is also used for purposes that other people are unaware of.

Baking soda rates right up there with hydrogen peroxide, which I always have in my medical drawer, as one of the most inexpensive and safe health tools around.

It wasn't until 1846 that Dr Austin Church and John Dwight began to manufacture and sell the compound we know as baking soda today. By the 1860s, baking soda featured in published cookbooks, and in the 1930s it was widely advertised as a "proven medical agent".

Baking soda taken internally (1 teaspoon in large glass of water) can help maintain the pH balance in your bloodstream, which could be why it has been recommended for use against both colds and influenza symptoms.

There is a fascinating article written about fighting the flu in 1918 and 1919 written by a doctor working with US Public Health Service. The doctor noticed that rarely anyone who had been thoroughly alkalised with bicarbonate of soda contracted the disease, and those who did contract it would invariably have mild attacks.

There are many ways to use the bicarb paste made with a little water, such as for sunburn, deodorant, splinter removal, plaque on teeth and gums, insect bites, teeth whitener, house cleaning, foot soak, exfoliator and powder added to the bath.

Baking soda mixed with white vinegar is a bubbly combination that has many uses. As a drain cleaner, sprinkle baking soda down the drain, then white/vinegar, and let it bubble for 15 minutes, then rinse with hot water.

I was amazed when I used it on my hand-basin drain, as I had avoided those other dreadful chemical drain cleaners which hadn't really worked. I think the blockage was mould.

Soak pots and pans in hot water and baking soda for 15 minutes to easily wipe away baked-on food.

Use baking soda to scrub your barbecue grill.

Baking soda can also be used as a fabric softener in your laundry or to get your clothes whither and brighter (add one cup to your laundry load).

Baking soda is a natural carpet cleaner. Sprinkle it onto carpets, let it sit for 15 minutes, then vacuum it up.

To polish silver without using toxic silver polish, fill your kitchen sink with hot water, add a sheet of aluminium foil and some baking soda and let the silver pieces soak until clean. It is an easy and fun way to clean silver.

Sprinkle baking soda in your shoes for a natural deodoriser.

You may find yourself inventing many other ways of using it.

In Italy, an oncologist by the name of Dr Simoncini uses baking soda or sodium bicarbonate for cancer treatment, mainly for the digestive tract. This includes cancers of the throat, colon, intestines, rectal area and other cancers in between. Cancers outside of the digestive tract generally need a health practitioner to inject the baking soda solution.

He has been persecuted in his own country, lost his medical licence and was threatened with jail, so I think he moved to another country. This shows that cancer is such a big business, with massive amounts of money spent on it that a near-costless cure is not accepted. What would they do with all those hospitals and clinics especially built?

Seems to be a few different ideas as to what cancer really is. Technically, cancer is caused by a bacterium inside cancer cells – not a fungus. However, some people think cancer is a fungus.

Alkalinity can kill these microbes and revert the cancer cells into normal cells.

If baking soda is taken daily, it may help reduce the destructive inflammation of autoimmune diseases like rheumatoid arthritis. This can encourage our spleen to create an anti-inflammatory environment that could be therapeutic in the face of inflammatory disease.

Baking soda and coconut oil, which is a skin regenerative, made into a paste and applied with a pad of cotton to basal cancer cells can heal. Be sure to soak the cotton-pad cover in vinegar prior to applying the paste with it. Tape it to the skin. This sort of skin cancer is not deadly, but it can spread on the skin if not totally cured.

Simple foods and substances around the home are used worldwide for medicines. These old folk remedies are finding newfound use now that science can validate their healing abilities with modern research.

When baking soda is combined with other safe and effective treatments like transdermal magnesium therapy, iodine, vitamin C and probiotics, cancers can be held at bay.

It is important to check the bicarb does not have aluminium in it. Our Australian McKenzie's bicarb is fine.

Apple cider vinegar 1/4 teaspoon and 1/4 teaspoon baking soda taken 2 times or more a day is another treatment. It can be done the same with lemon and baking soda, or lime and baking soda formulas.

Bicarb soda recipe – by mouth to alkalise – my version:

25% bicarb

75% maple syrup

a little warm water to mix.

From what I understand, maple syrup is the only sweet food that is alkaline. It cleared up my dermatitis when I used it 3 times a day.

Women can take 1–4 teaspoons in water, morning and night, for urgent alkalising, men up to 6–8 per day. This is according to an old friend who had been a nurse and self cured.

Perhaps honey could be substituted for maple syrup for those who live where there is none. I think I read somewhere that using molasses with the bicarb worked for these people.

It is useful to keep you feeling you are doing the right thing by using a pH (acidity) tape and that it shows well over 5, preferably 7 or 8, to avoid illness. Five is the borderline of acidity to stay healthy. You can get pH tape for testing at health-food shops.

There is nothing like a hot soak in a magnesium-chloride bath with bicarbonate before bed. Such soaks are heaven on earth for people who suffer from insomnia and feelings of restlessness in the limbs.

Use Epsom salts and magnesium chloride bath flakes (equal amounts).

BEES

Without them, we would die. Bees are of great importance as they support most growth in fruit and vegetables.

People are now working out how to pollinate without bees because so many are dying from all the toxins we spray around, along with radiation waves. It has been reported that 5G killed a hive once it was turned on.

Bee pollen is an important substance and is sometimes called a superfood as it possesses all of the nutrients essential to sustain human life, with a breakdown of 55% carbohydrates, 35% protein, 3% vitamins and minerals, 2% fatty acids and 5% other substances.

Many bodybuilders and Olympic athletes use bee pollen to increase strength and endurance, and it is also effective in decreasing recovery time after workouts.

Having been a great user of honey instead of sugar since early childhood, I was fascinated to learn more about what was used from the bees, such as pollen on its own and bee propolis in foods, healthy products and much more. I have only discovered this in recent years.

Whenever I feel sort of funny in the throat, as if a cold or illness is on the way, I squirt propolis in the back of my mouth. Certainly haven't had a cold or infection.

It is the yellow crunchy top of the honey that can be made into ointment, sweets and more. This part of the honey has been found to have a healing effect on just about anything you can think of, including burns. It also prevents dental cavities and genital herpes.

I buy an ointment, Bright's, which includes jojoba, and find it clears warts, itches, little cancer cells, bruises, some acne and anything on my skin.

Propolis doesn't just benefit bees (coating their hives to prevent parasites), it has been used for thousands of years as folk medicine. Some uses were as bee glue to treat abscesses, heal wounds and fight infection. In fact, propolis was listed as an official drug in the London pharmacopoeias of the 17th century.

BLACK

Black is the colour of death and depression. It is also used for authority. Black is secretive, withholding and hot due to absorbing heat, whereas white is an out flowing, fresh and cooling expression. My black doormat on the balcony can be boiling hot but the pale grey tiles underneath are just warm.

Now whole suburbs are black and greys instead of the cooler colours of the past. They are now proving to be much hotter too. As most trees cut down.

Today people wear it to the gym or dance class. You look slimmer, but lycra is holding everything in. It doesn't breathe or release energy and toxins. At yoga, they used to say wear loose clothing. Don't think too many do that now.

Nearly all organisations' uniforms (including small rural businesses in the northern part of Australia and inland where it is hot) are black with a coloured logo to differentiate from others and it can only be read up close and even harder if I haven't got my glasses on.

Really sorry for the firies now in black, except for their bright jackets. Even the barman on a luxury yacht in black. Why weren't they wearing sea blue or green to put you in the mood? Uniforms used to be designed with the colours of the business as the banks did in the past. Colours give you the feeling of the organisation.

Black is also the colour, along with dark brown, of Capricorn. Few Capricorns look good in it, except those with red hair or white blonde like Marlene Dietrich. My recent idea is that, now Pluto has left Capricorn after 20 years and is in Aquarius, we may gradually start wearing more bright, powerful colours

Queen Victoria wore it for 10 years after her husband died. Normally, widows were expected to wear black for a year after death of a husband and were not to marry again until after then.

Only up to a few years ago did women after child bearing wear black from head to toe (always with stockings as well) in Greece and Italy. Obviously, so they wouldn't be attractive or attracted to other men. No one looks pretty or romantic in black.

As time went on, Coco Chanel almost caused an uproar by wearing what is now known as the "little black dress". However, it is highlighted by great jewellery (Audrey Hepburn) or flowing colour scarfs or flowers and of course with white.

This was primarily for after-5 chic. Today it is almost uniform across the board. Really feel sorry to see brides and bridesmaids wearing it. Doesn't have to be white, but some other colour would be more positive. In India, the bride wears red. A friend of mine wore red and had everyone else in white. Looked great.

BLOOD
– see "O"

Blood types – see "O" the diet of the Hunter Gatherer (my type)

There are books out on blood-type diet, such as "**Live Right for Your Type**" by Peter D'Adamo. I have found that using my O diet is very successful.

This was easy at first, as I had to give up several foods but did it gradually. Now I follow my correct food but occasionally, or when I am on holidays or out (like an art show opening),

I wallow in cheese which is not for O type and other foods with wheat. Have to say I use goat/sheep cheese and yoghurt at times. Soft cheeses are less acidic than hard ones. I think my basic intake of food is good for me so the other food has little effect. Also, I suggest (and forget) to say, "Everything I eat makes me happy and healthy".

Look up the internet for blood types. You will find the Food Most Beneficial. Food Allowed and Food not Allowed. It seems that some foods will be the reason for weight loss or gain.

Bleeding

At one time in my life, I found myself suddenly bleeding badly, even during periods, and having an operation to stop it. Couldn't keep doing that so checked in with my natural therapist and, along with herbal mixture, he suggested I needed to strengthen my reproduction area by using sitz baths every day for about 3 months,

In the old days they made a special bath for people to sit in with comfort. I believe Churchill used one.

Most convenient for me was a baby bath, filled in the shower and sat with my feet outside the shower in slippers or on a mat.

If cold, I kept a warm top on, tucked into my bra. Cold water draws blood to the area for healing circulation. One way of reading a lot of good books.

Dysfunctional bleeding

I went through some years of dysfunctional bleeding on and off. Usually bought about by extremely emotional situations and often round February, which is when the full moon is usually closest to the earth. Hospitals and police only a few years back called it the bleeding/crazy season.

Homeopathic pills or a medicine I could get mixed by a naturopath would stop it in a very short time.

Blood pressure chart

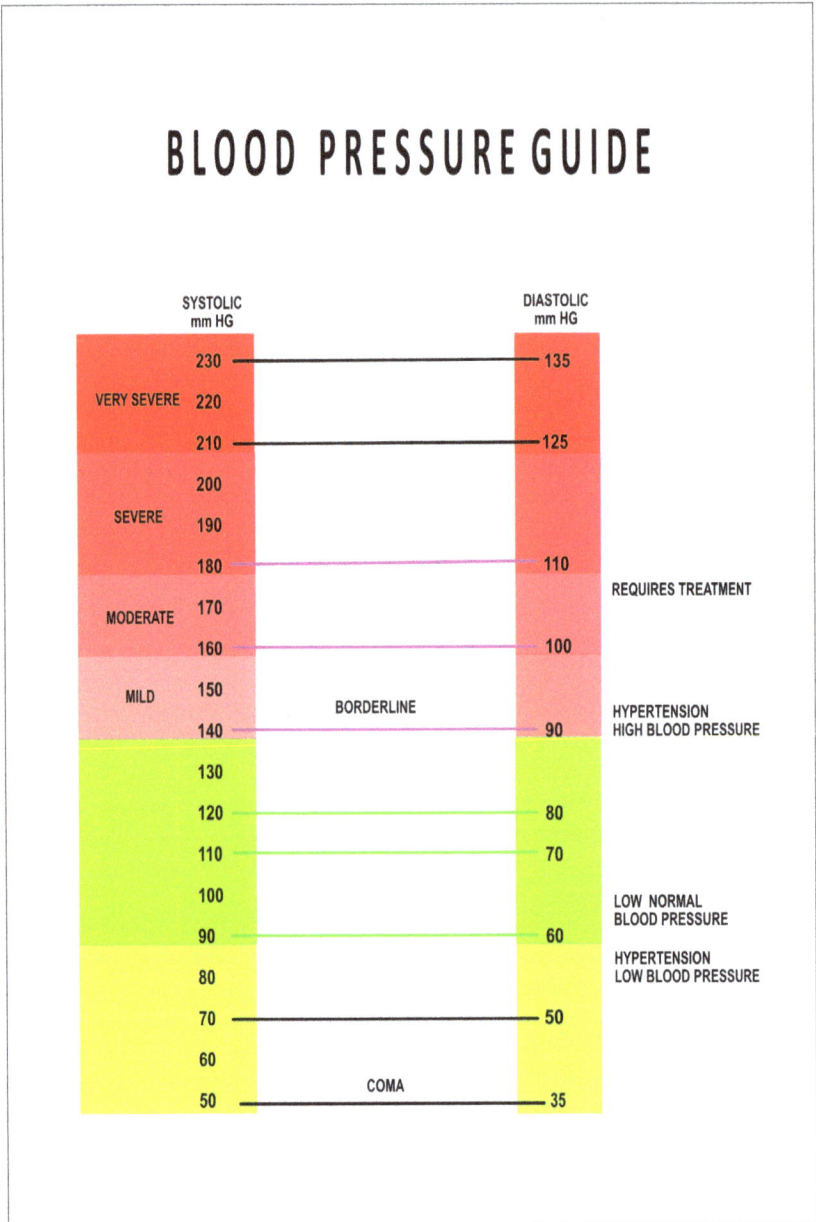

BRAIN

There are many books out regarding the brain's elasticity. An excellent one is by Bessel van der Kolk called ***The Body Keeps the Score: Brain, Mind, and Body in the Healing of Trauma***. The author shows how the brain connects with so many health problems.

Brain Damage – Ready to turn off the machine in the hospital – be patient.

Using 20 gm a day of omega 3 oil intravenously can turn a person around and within a year back to normal.

How to keep young

I'm sure many of you have read articles in Style Manual on how to stay young. Use the muscle between your ears in many ways every day. Do things such as:

Cut down sugar intake by using almonds, berries, etc.

Go ballroom dancing and any other kind of dancing.

Go walking for at least 20 minutes.

Take vitamins and minerals that are good for the brain.

Volunteer to answer questions at the library, museum, hospital, etc.

Play video games – not for too long, as the radiation is not good for you.

Complete jig saws, cross words and any other puzzles.

Leave your comfort zone.

Avoid stress with mediation.

Really listen to details.

Drink herbal teas – try sage and rosemary (great for memory).

Attend classes at local library, seminars and other educational events.

Sing – join a choir even if you think you're no good.

Listen to music.

Eat fish and any seafood – they are very good for us, especially tinned sardines.

Choose a sport side so you can get stirred up but not angry, which is bad for you.

Talk business and politics – debating is good for you and helps formulate your thoughts.

Sleep – do all you can to get good sleep, and a siesta sleep is always a great way of recharging, I find.

Join a book club – good socially but also stirs the brain.

Massage – stretch your neck and roll your shoulders to help the nerves to the brain.

Read the news to keep up with what is happening locally or in the world.

Learn to play a musical instrument.

Avoid electromagnetic radiation as much as possible – use the phone on loudspeaker.

Brain surgeon Dr Charlie Teo's advice

Protection is mainly why electricals, especially in the bedrooms, should be turned off completely when not in use. Also, microwaved foods should not be eaten immediately. Wait a few minutes as the food continues to be cooked after it has been taken out of the oven.

Dr Charlie Teo (from Australia's Channel 7's Last Chance Surgery) says it's better to avoid electromagnetic radiation.

Dr Charlie Teo has urged people to put mobile phones on loudspeaker, move clock radios to the foot of the bed and wait until microwaves have finished beeping before opening them.

The controversial Sydney specialist told a Melbourne fundraiser that although the jury was still out on mobile phones and other forms of electromagnetic radiation, we should not take risks. "Even though the jury's not in, just to err on the side of safety, I would try and limit the amount of electromagnetic radiation that you're exposed to", he said.

"The American government, for example, recommend that all electrical appliances should be put at the foot of the bed and not the head of the bed."

"Electric blankets should be turned off before you get in bed and definitely wait for those 5 beeps before you open the microwave."

"With the mobile phone, I encourage you to put it on loudspeaker and step outside rather than sticking it up to your brain."

Dr Teo, who tackles tumours other surgeons deem inoperable, said some hair dyes, particularly red, could also cause brain cancer in people with a predisposition.

"The body needs some genetic predisposition. The hair dye, the mobile phone, they're just catalysts but you probably need some sort of genetic aberration to get the cancer in the first place", he said.

BREATHING
– see Diabetes

It is suggested to do yogic alternating nostril breathing every day. Hold one side of the nose closed, then breathe in and breathe out the other side while holding down the nostril you just breathed in with. It helps restore imbalances in your brain – improves sleep – calms your emotional state – boosts your thinking – calms your nervous system.

You don't breathe through them equally all the time. Right now, you will be favouring either your left nostril or your right nostril. Left nostril is for calming – right nostril for energy.

Your nose is directly linked to your brain and nervous system. For thousands of years the Indian yogis have believed that many diseases are connected to disturbed nasal breathing.

Another good, relaxing activity involves slow conscious breathing where you breathe slowly into the abdomen (tummy breathing), exhale even more slowly and then, when fully exhaled, hold the breath until the urge to breathe is triggered. Try to hold your breath for longer. This is not good if there is a heart problem.

So many of us are shallow breathers, so we don't get all the oxygen we need to be healthy.

Don't hold your breath at any time if you have high blood pressure.

Today the most unlikely people will say breathe in deeply and out slowly if someone is stressing out. Now taken for granted that breathing helps calm. It is easy to take breathing for granted, because we don't have to think about it. Only when we do are we reminded of its importance, and most times, the reminder is forced by getting out of breath climbing the stairs and similar situations.

BURNS

Healing burns

There are many ways of healing burns that people have discovered, but most people don't know or think about it but need to be used ASAP.

Egg whites on the burn. May use all the eggs you've got. Leave it on as long as possible but it has proved to work

Cold water. Plunge the arm or leg straight into a bucket of cold water. I'll never forget seeing a photo of someone who had instinctively plunged the arm in the bucket of water. The water didn't go all the way up and there was a very bad scar where it hadn't been in the water. Otherwise, the rest was fine.

Cold water stops the continual burning, so some do the water and then the egg whites.

This treatment for burns is used for teaching beginner firemen. First aid consists of first spraying cold water on the affected area until the heat is reduced, which stops the continued burning of all layers of the skin. Then, spread the egg whites onto the affected area.

Sticking your hand into a bowl of flour for 10 minutes. An ex-Vietnam soldier said when he was on fire, they threw a bag of flour all over him to put the fire out. Not only put the fire out, but he never even had a blister!!!!

It is suggested you put a bag of flour in the fridge in case, as it feels better than room temperature.

Reiki heals if you can use it on the area immediately or someone else can use it on you. In my experience, it prevents blisters and completely heals as it did with a close friend who had a habit of lifting her baking dishes and forgetting to use the glove. When I held her hand between my hands, she wanted to pull away and do something else, but I hung on until it cooled and she was amazed to find she had no new scar among the others.

BUTTER

Butter v. margarine

Margarine was developed for other purposes, but it was decided to also make a spread. It was a pale grey/white with no appeal, so they put colour in and sold it as butter replacement. Both have more or less the same calories. Butter has, however, many nutritional benefits, whereas margarine has what has been added. Butter tastes better and improves the flavour. Margarine doesn't.   If you prefer you can use Ghee which is a form of butter used in Indian cooking.

Margarine is but ONE MOLECULE away from being PLASTIC and shares 27 ingredients with PAINT, which is of course is not told to the public.

I was into margarine for a short time and then the olive-oil spread they put out to replace butter. However, always preferred butter, and when I read about how good for you it is, I stuck with it. Obviously too much butter, like anything else, can cause problems. It is a diary food, which many avoid. Organic is best.

A few years ago, a friend suggested I buy a tub of margarine and leave it open on the front step in the sun for a week. I was amazed to note over the time that nothing happened. It just looked like the same perfect tub. Obviously, no bugs or creature was tempted. In other words, indigestible.

What happens to our poor bodies when we have eaten that? Margarine must be put in the fridges in the supermarket to kid you, but it doesn't have a smelt.

C

CALCIUM

– see Osteoporosis

I received an article in an email with some comments about 2 sisters in Holland who had osteoporosis. One went down the medical road and felt no better in a year, whereas the other did what is shown below with egg shells and was fine.

For myself, 10 years before I was diagnosed with osteoporosis, my doctor told me to take hormone replacement therapy, as my bone density was low, and if I didn't, I would be in a wheelchair in 10 years. I haven't been in a wheelchair yet and feel quite well.

Once I was diagnosed about 10 years later, I didn't want to take any of the drugs. So, I proceeded to keep to much more alkaline foods, as acids collect in the bones, and I did more exercise and took various other things like almonds, calcium, etc.

I don't use dairy due to my O-blood-type style of food. (In fact, my first osteopath when I was a child told us not to drink milk as it caused mucus. I suffered from bronchitis at the time). I avoided more testing until a new doctor wanted to test my bone density again, so I decided I might as well see what had been going on over the past 6 years. I had never had a broken bone and don't have any pain.

For some time before that (can't remember how long) I had been following the process below. After my test, I rang the doctor to see how things were. The receptionist asked me what I wanted. I told her and she came back saying all was fine. I didn't continue with the eggshells (below) after a while.

Recently, after 5 years, I had a scan and now have osteoporosis again. So back to the egg shells and of course other foods. Too much calcium can cause trouble by bunching up into lumps.

How to make your own super calcium supplement?

Wash some empty eggshells in warm water and let them dry. I collect quite a few in a glass jar and put in the fridge and keep going until its full and ready to grind.

Break them into small pieces and grind them into a fine powder. Coffee grinders work best, but a blender or even a mortar and pestle will do. Store the powder in an airtight GLASS jar in the fridge.

Mix ½ - 1 teaspoon of powdered eggshell with the juice of half a freshly squeezed lemon. The solution will start to bubble and foam. (I use an egg cup to do this).

Leave at room temperature for at least 6 hours and that's it! Ready to take.

(I'm too impatient to wait more than 6 hours). Do this once a day.

Half a teaspoon of eggshell gives you about 400 mg of calcium citrate, which is the recommended amount you should take each day.

Most Asian, African, South American, and tribal people don't use dairy and rarely seem to suffer from osteoporosis. What do they eat or not eat? Non-acidic food and probably do more exercise.

A handful of almonds also gives you your day's worth of calcium.

CANCER

 – see – Bicarb soda, Baking soda, Coconut oil, EMF, Ginger, Hemp oil, Fruit, Milk, Salves, Mushrooms, Cinnamon, Curcumin (turmeric), Celery, Cloves, Lemon, Pawpaw and Pineapple.

Alternative cancer treatments

After years of oncologists telling people chemotherapy is the only way to try ('try' being the key word) to eliminate cancer, patients are still dying by the thousands each year. Even pharmacists and doctors who handle and dispense these toxic chemicals are getting cancer at a much higher rate than the general population. There is an alternative way.

Causes of cancer can be:

Electricity – Electromagnetic field (EMF) – due to electronic equipment and dirty electricity which used to be delivered at 50 Hz but now much more. Touch lights are very bad. Where you sleep there should be no television, electrical things in the bedroom – or at least at the foot of the bed. Feng shui would agree with this. Bedrooms are only for making love and sleeping. They did a test with 1,200 fluorescent tubes standing upright under power lines, not attached to any switches or wires, and they all lit up.

Stress – Worrying is using your imagination to create something you don't want. People put wealth before health and it is not worth it. Organic food may be more expensive, but it cost thousands to go through chemo, etc. Using 80% organic reduces pesticides in urine by 90%. Malnutrition also causes obesity.

Water – Hydration. This needs to be high-quality water. Hydration gets the nutrients to the cells giving the gut-viable bacteria. Drinking lots of water doesn't mean you are getting hydrated. Often the body doesn't absorb it. Use a little sea salt in to help absorb.

We need to eliminate the primary causes of cancer. We may seem to be doing everything right but not feeling right. What stops it? Check the condition, look for blockages, emotional and physical. Disease is a warning system.

Some other causes – Mould, parasites, heavy metals, yeast which can be found in air-con and car air con, etc. Radiation (EMF) is the primary intolerance, also fungus, bacteria and food intolerances.

Sleep – I find 6 hours okay, but generally don't get it. Chinese medicine says go to bed between 9 and 11.

We are beings of light, operating with millions of light cells which are all affected by these things.

Fermented food is very good for you as it was always used where refrigeration wasn't available. Sauerkraut is extremely good. Also kimchi.

You will find in the References page at the back organisations specialising in retreats, workshops and counselling

for healing cancer and other ailments, including spiritual, emotional and physical problems.

There are probably many more, but these are the ones I know of.

Cancer Tips

Every person has cancer cells in the body. These cancer cells do not show up in the standard tests until they have multiplied to a few billion. When doctors tell cancer patients that there are no more cancer cells in their bodies after treatment, it just means the tests are unable to detect the cancer cells because they have not reached the detectable size.

When the person's immune system is strong, the cancer cells will be destroyed and prevented from multiplying and forming tumours.

Chemotherapy involves poisoning the rapidly growing cancer cells and destroys rapidly growing healthy cells in the bone marrow, gastro-intestinal tract, etc., and can cause organ damage, such as in liver, kidneys, heart, lungs, etc. Any treatment that makes a sick person sicker cannot be good.

Radiation, while destroying cancer cells, also burns, scars and damages healthy cells, tissues, and organs.

Initial treatment with chemotherapy and radiation will often reduce tumour size. However, prolonged use of chemotherapy and radiation do not result in more tumour destruction.

What many people aren't aware of is that chemotherapy and radiation can cause cancer cells to mutate and become resistant and difficult to destroy. Surgery can also cause cancer cells to spread to other sites.

Of course, these do heal many people, though often it comes back, as it has for several of my friends, and are all very painful.

I think that an effective way to battle cancer is to starve the cancer cells by not feeding them with the foods they need to multiply.

Cancer cells feed on sugar and salt. Cut them off as much as possible and don't use the chemical sweeteners. Instead use maple syrup, Manuka honey or molasses, but only in very small amounts. Table salt has a chemical added to make it white in colour. Better alternatives are natural Himalayan, river salts and sea salt. They contain a lot of good minerals.

Milk causes the body to produce mucus, especially in the gastro-intestinal tract. Cancer feeds on mucus. By cutting off milk and substituting with fresh fruit juice, nut milks, cancer cells are being starved. Throw some nuts in a blender with some water and make your own nut milk.

Cancer cells thrive in an acid environment. When your pH reaches 4.0, you're headed for real trouble. A meat-based diet is acidic, though O-blood people need meat. It is a good idea to eat fish and less meat (organic), as the usual meat also contains livestock antibiotics, growth hormones and parasites, which are all harmful.

A diet made of 80% fresh vegetables (steamed, stir-fried or baked) and juice can be boring at first but do it slowly, and you will gradually find you enjoy it. Use whole grains, seeds, nuts, and a little fruit to help put the body into an alkaline environment. About 20% can be from cooked food, including beans.

To obtain live enzymes for building healthy cells, try and drink fresh vegetable juice (most vegetables including bean sprouts) and eat some raw vegetables 2 or 3 times a day (at least eat some during the day).

Avoid or reduce consumption of coffee, tea, and chocolate, which have high caffeine. Green tea is a better alternative and has cancer-fighting properties, and dark 75% chocolate is OK.

Water – best to drink purified water or filtered, to avoid known toxins and heavy metals in tap water. Purified water needs to be used also for cooking, making ice and so on. Add some lemon if you don't like the taste of water.

Meat protein is difficult to digest and requires a lot of digestive enzymes. Undigested meat remaining in the intestines becomes putrefied and leads to more toxic build up.

Cancer is a disease of the mind, body, and spirit. A proactive and positive spirit will help the cancer warrior to be a survivor. Anger, unwillingness to forgive, resentment and bitterness put the body into a stressful and acidic environment. Learn to have a loving and forgiving spirit. Relax and enjoy life.

Exercising daily and deep breathing help to get more oxygen down to the cellular level. Oxygen therapy is another means to destroy cancer cells.

Do not put:

plastic containers in microwave

water bottles in freezer

plastic wrap in microwave.

Food should be put in glass or ceramic containers where possible. Much safer to use tempered glass, Pyrex or Corning Ware, etc. If using the microwave (which kills life), put a paper towel instead of plastic wrap, which when heated is poisonous.

These are some cures I've read about:

A man diagnosed with stage-4 prostate cancer was told that sudden pH surges destroy cancer. He ordered caesium, but it didn't arrive in time for his next medical examination. Instead, he tried pH purging with bicarbonate of soda and molasses. In weeks, he was cancer free.

A concerned father sneaked tetrahydrocannabinol (THC) hemp oil into his toddler son's feeding tube to reverse his ebbing health during cancer treatments. The little boy's health surged, and he became cancer free. The doctors never knew what the father did to reverse the boy's failing health.

A middle-aged New Zealand man with leukaemia went into a coma from flu/pneumonia complications. The hospital staff threatened to pull his life support until the family members insisted they try mega-dose intravenous vitamin C. He walked out of the hospital days later. A year later, his check-up showed that he was now leukaemia free.

Environmental and lifestyle factors are increasingly being pinpointed as the primary culprits fuelling our cancer epidemic. These include:

Pesticide and other chemical exposures, processed and artificial foods (plus the chemicals in the packaging), wireless technologies, dirty electricity, and medical diagnostic radiation exposure, pharmaceutical drugs, obesity, stress and poor sleeping habits. Lack of sunshine exposure and use of sunscreens.

Cancer-fighting superfoods:

Garlic, onions, leeks, shallots, and chives

These all help to regulate blood sugar levels

Green tea

Is an antioxidant and helps the liver cleanse.

Cruciferous vegetables

Cabbages, sprouts, broccoli, and cauliflower contain powerful anti-cancer molecules.

Mushrooms

Mushrooms stimulate the reproduction of immune cells

Turmeric

The most powerful natural anti-inflammatory identified today. To be assimilated by the body, turmeric needs to be mixed with black pepper. I take a teaspoon of powder, one of honey, each morning with lemon juice and warm water.

Fruits and vegetables rich in carotenoids

Carrots, yams, sweet potatoes, squash, tomatoes, apricots, beets and all the brightly coloured fruits and vegetables contain vitamin A and lycopene, which have the proven capacity to inhibit the growth of particularly aggressive cancers.

Herbs and spices

Rosemary, thyme, oregano, basil and mint are rich in essential oils.

Carotenoids

Multiple studies demonstrate that vitamin A and carotenoids help in the prevention and treatment of many cancers in a variety of ways.

Citrus fruit

Oranges, tangerines, lemons and grapefruit contain anti-inflammatory.

Dandelion

It has been used by traditional medical systems all over the world for digestive, kidney, liver, and spleen disorders, as well as tumours of the lung, breast, and uterus. Use the tea.

Review your lifestyle as preventative measures against the development of cancer. Existing cancers may stop growing, or grow more slowly.

Breast cancer – see Milk, Pomegranate.

Personally, I think underwire bras can be one of the reasons for breast cancer.

In case you haven't read about this before, bra-free women have about the same incidence of breast cancer as men, while the incidence rises the tighter and longer the bra is worn.

It has to do with constriction of the lymphatic system within the breasts caused by tight bras, resulting in fluid and toxin accumulation. This can lead to cysts, pain, and tissue toxi-fication, and ultimately may result in cancer. Before wired bras, there was a lot less breast cancer.

Some may remember the trauma at the ABC in Brisbane where so many were going down with cancer. Many people now think the constant connection with electronic wires, etc. coming up through their legs and around caused the energy to enter the underwire bras. Great reading on the subject is by Donna Fisher – **More Silent Fields: Cancer and the dirty electricity plague**.

Another concern for people who are following up breast cancer in their own way is the electric blanket. Lying on the side the breast rests on the wiring. It is suggested you warm the bed up and turn it off and unplug from the electrical socket.

Skin cancer – see Aloe Vera, Chick weed. Dandelion is excellent to apply for skin cancers.

Salve (black salve)

Black salve is an escharotic, from the Greek word which means "to burn", made of a combination of 4 different herbs (bloodroot, galangal, chaparral and graviola) in a solution of zinc chloride. The resulting paste, which is a very dark brown colour, when put on a spot where cancer cells are present, will go through the layer of skin to reach the cancer cells, kill and enclose the malignant cells in what looks like a black scab.

The tissue surrounding the scab may look slightly inflamed with a white circle of pus around the scab. After 7 to 10 days the scab will fall off, leaving a clean healthy wound where the cancer was. The wound will then quickly heal and fill up with new healthy cells in a very short time.

I was fascinated when I did it once. Think I put a band aid over it but not sure. It left a circular hole red round the edges and sort of watery inside. As it healed, I used **Rosa scarless healer cream.**

Black salve has also been successfully used to treat other types of cancers and several testimonials can be found on webpages.

Warning: The Therapeutic Goods Administration (TGA) does not approve the sale of black salve for use on people, so this product is "For Animal Use Only". However, the ingredients and their amount are the same.

CANDIDA

I found staying off anything related to yeast for 3 months helped clear candida. You can easily find yeast-free bread now, and preferably not made with wheat. Sadly, wine has yeast in it. Strawberries can have mould, similarly, with mushrooms, blue cheese, etc. For sugar, use Stevia or maple syrup instead.

For the last 30 years, I've done my best to have yeast-free bread and other yeast-type foods. Now sourdough is quite common, which is much better for you.

I also kept off wine (don't drink beer) for the 3 months but gin and vodka are distilled, so okay to drink with tonic or similar, not with fruit flavour – too much sugars. Fresh lemon should be OK.

THRUSH is cleared with a tea-tree oil douche. 500 ml of warm water with as much tea-tree (sting) as you can stand. Start with a couple of teaspoons.

Using a teaspoon of bicarb soda in water by mouth daily will help clear candida internally.

These of course aren't the only cures, but they have worked for me.

CANNABIS – hemp

Cannabis extract medicine, also known as "hemp oil" is a concentrated formulation of cannabis that is ingested orally.

The cannabinoids are much more concentrated than with smoking, so it has a more powerful effect on your system.

The oil is ingested, not smoked, meaning it is digested through the system that is meant to absorb nutrients.

Essentially, you are feeding your body the pure molecules that enable it to stay balanced, and since all disease is an imbalance of some kind, this medicine is effective against nearly anything. At least, that's what the bulk of science and real experience show.

Cannabis sativa hemp, the miracle plant, contains the cure for cancer and other ailments.   It is an ancient medicine.

The current restrictions against hemp were put in place and maintained, not because hemp is evil or harmful, but for big money to make more big money, while we suffer and die needlessly. Look at a proposal such as this: if we were allowed to grow hemp in our back yards and cure our own illnesses, what do you think the reaction of the pharmaceutical industry would be to such a plan?

Pharmaceutical companies that still exist today sold hemp-based medicines in the 1800s and early 1900s.

Uses of medical marijuana

Aside from recreational use, there are as many as 14 applications for medical marijuana. Here are some of them:

minimising seizures

nausea relief

pain relief

delaying first signs of Alzheimer's.

There is a lot of information on the internet as it has now been approved by the government. However, some people find the limited amount not enough to stop the pain, etc. They want a stronger one, and not as expensive either.

CELL SALTS

There are 12 cell salts developed by Dr Schuessler over 150 years ago

These are available in health-food shops and some chemists. They cover all the areas and problems in the body. Inexpensive, tasteless and no side effects. Just chew them to be absorbed into your system, bypassing the liver.

One of my favourites is mag phos, which is a muscle relaxant and fixes cramp in no time. You can take as much as you like when having a cramp.

Astrologers allocate them to star signs.

Cell salts (abbreviated) and astrology

FIRE	EARTH	AIR	WATER
ARIES	CAPRICORN	LIBRA	CANCER
Ruler – Mars	Ruler – Saturn	Ruler –Venus	Ruler – Moon
Kali phos	Calc phos	Nat phos	Calc flur
Stress, headaches, nervous tension	Fatigue, sore throat	Indigestion, gas, hyperacidity	Colds, chaffed skin, haemorrhoids
LEO	TAURUS	AQUARIUS	SCORPIO
Ruler – Sun	Ruler – Venus	Ruler – Uranus	Ruler – Pluto
Mag phos	Nat sulph	Nat mur	Calc sulph
Muscle cramps & pain	Flu, vomiting, nausea	Colds, headaches, dizziness	Acne, colds, sore throat
SAGITTARIUS	VIRGO	GEMINI	PISCES
Ruler – Jupiter	Ruler – Mercury	Ruler –Mercury	Ruler – Neptune
Silica	Kali sulph	Kali mur	Ferr phos
Brittle hair & nails, skin eruptions	Cold, skin eruptions	Colds, sore throats, runny nose	Fevers, colds, minor sweating

CHARCOAL

Many years ago, a friend was rushed to hospital for his appendix. After, he was having a lot of pain in the gut. His father brought in some charcoal tablets for the pain (wind). The nurse was so pleased to see it. She said, "They always used it in the past but not anymore".

CHAKRAS

Today, most people are familiar with the word and meaning of "chakras". They also have colours indicating the energy. These can be used on the area of pain to ease the problem, though of course it can be over used.

First	Second	Third	Fourth	Fifth	Sixth	Seventh
Red	Orange	Yellow	Green	Blue	Indigo	Purple

CHEMOTHERAPY

– see Cancer, Death

The US and UK governments killed 1.5 million people in Iraq, based on lies about weapons of mass destruction they knew did not exist. The medical/pharmaceutical world kills more than that every year – and seems to be is even more corrupt than the political/governmental world.

Many chemo drugs are listed as "a known carcinogen", and those applying it must be tested on a regular basis as many of them get cancer.

Yes, chemo may shrink a tumour, but it can make cancer come back stronger in particular. It often creates the secondaries that kill you 2 years later.

A friend of mine was taking the oral chemo after in-hospital chemo and radiation. She was to take it for 6 months but was becoming more and more unwell so stopped after 2 months. Many months later she said, "If I had continued it, I would be dead now".

CHI

Chi chart

TIME	SLEEP EXERCISE	BODY	ACTION
5 – 7 am Yang	Rub flesh between finger and thumb	Large intestine	Drink water, stretch, meditate and exercise
7 – 9 am Ying	Tap under the eyes	Stomach	Breakfast, be kind to self
9 – 11 am Yang	Circular pressure over spleen	Spleen	Make decisions, work hard, think, communicate
11 am – 1 pm Ying	Rub armpit area	Heart	Articulate vision, access soul, spread the love
1 – 3 pm Yang	Deep pressure around	Small intestine	Lunch, go slow
3 – 5 pm Ying	Rub area on nose between eyes	Bladder	Go with the flow, cruise

5 – 7 pm Yang	Rub centre behind ball ball of big toe	Kidneys	Switch off, share a laugh, sex, acknowledge skill
7 – 9 pm Ying	Massage middle finger	Pericardium	Come home, dinner, sex
9 – 11 pm Yang	Rub behind your ears	San Jiao	Go to bed, go to sleep
11 – 1 am Ying	Rub above your ears	Gall bladder	Sleep
1 – 3 am Yang	Rub area over liver	Liver	Sleep
3 – 5 am Ying	Rub between upper arms and shoulder	Lungs	Embody your dreams

In recent years, I have had spells of dizziness, nausea, no energy and even fainted once, which I put down to low blood sugar. I call it my "wonky day" and when mild I just lie around doing Reiki and sleep.

The doctors gave me all sorts of tests but couldn't come up with anything. So naturally I went to acupuncture. Simple, I had imbalance of chi, ying and yang. Sometimes he says the chi is stagnant. After a treatment, I'm off and running. We still can't work out what causes it.

CHIA SEED

Herbalists, healers are always coming up with something new that is good for us, which is great.

What began in South America has taken off in Australia, and John Foss is now the world's largest producer of Chia seed.

In modern-day medicine, omega 3 is well known for its prevention of heart disease and strokes.

Chia seed was used by the Aztecs and now, more recently Australia has recognised the dietary benefits of chia. It has only recently been re-discovered. Chia is described as nature's multivitamin.

I use it in porridge, though many sprinkle it on their salad or smoothie. It can block up in areas of the body that we are unaware of as they are so tiny. It can take a while to find out what the problem is, so don't use too many raw ones unless widely sprinkled. I soak mine in the porridge before I go out for a walk, then cook so it digests.

CHILLI

Chillies are an excellent source of vitamins A, B, C and E, with minerals like molybdenum, manganese, folate, potassium, thiamine, and copper. Chilli contains 7 times more vitamin C than orange.

Ever since their introduction to India in 1498, chillies have been included in Ayurvedic medicines and used as a tonic to ward off many diseases. Chillies are good for slimming down as they easily burn calories. They stimulate the appetite and digestive system, as well as help clear the lungs.

Chillies have antioxidants that can lower cholesterol. High cholesterol can cause illnesses such as atherosclerosis, heart disease, cataracts, osteoarthritis and rheumatoid arthritis. Chillies also dilate the airways, which reduces asthma and wheezing.

Chillies can be used in various forms to act as a detoxicant, pain killer and anti-inflammatory. They can help with cancer, heart attack and lung disease.

Benefits of using chilli in food include:

- beautiful skin and improved circulation

- relief and prevention of arthritis – offers pain relief and is anti-inflammatory

- lowered blood pressure, enhanced circulatory system and maintenance of strong cell walls

- relief for cluster headaches and migraines – rub a chilli on your temples

- reduced flu symptoms, sinusitis, respiratory problems and muscle pain
- dried psoriasis patches – use topical capsicum creams
- ulcer relief
- improved libido and sex drive.

CHINESE MEDICINE

This form of prevention and healing has been developed over thousands of years. Therefore, it is one of the recommended forms of healing.

I find at different times I mix and match all kinds of healing, depending on what seems to be working at the time. Often, I use a physical form of healing, massage, acupuncture, etc. along with an internal one such as herbal, homeopathic, or Chinese medicine.

Slapping used in Chinese Medicine.

This can indicate that something is wrong – if you get inflamed or painful in a certain area – and it's good for circulation.

Slap shoulders, joints first, then arm with right hand on elbow turned up. This heals or shows up heart, cholesterol, etc. Slap hard the knees when sitting, stand to hit behind them, then top of hands (good for constipation), tops of feet by bringing up to rest on a chair or cross to other leg to slap under.

Hands and feet are the ends of the meridians.

Slapping lets the ying out as the yang rises and warms the body. Activates your own healing.

CHOLESTEROL

CLEANSE RECIPE 1

Probably good for general cleansing too.

This simple, natural and effective 7-week program will restore healthy levels of cholesterol throughout the cardiovascular system.

Prepare

30 cloves of garlic (peeled)

5–6 (depending on size) diced (cut up) fresh lemons including rind (not peeled)

Mince these in a blender or food processor.

Place in a saucepan with 1 litre of water.

Then bring to the boil but DO NOT BOIL.

Strain well, let it cool and bottle in glass containers and keep in the fridge, lasts for 3 weeks.

Treatment

Take a daily dose of 30 ml (only) before or after the main meal of the day. Do this for 3 weeks.

After the 3 weeks, have a 7-day break.

Then repeat the process for another 3 weeks.

This is a cheap, safe and therapeutic course of treatment. It is recommended that it be repeated once a year.

CLEANSE RECIPE 2 – see Tamarind

Recommended by my naturopath (less complicated). This is the one I used and was amazed how my cholesterol went down in a few months.

CIRCUMCISION

Some doctors are concerned about the falling circumcision rates as they are putting baby boys at risk of health problems for both men and women.

Of course, because circumcision is performed on a sexual organ, it causes emotional and religious debate. The fact that the Jews used it (sadly a giveaway during the Second World War) made sense to me as, living in the Middle East, it would have been for health reasons, the same with, I think, the banning of pork and milk as part of the religious way of life related to health.

There are arguments that can be made on the good and bad sides. When uncircumcised, men are more likely to get penile cancer, urinary tract infections, sexually transmitted diseases (STDs), ulcers and human papillomavirus (HPV) which can be in the genitalia of both sexes

In the warmer climates in Australia, there are more circumcised babies. Tasmania has the least.

Young men in late teens are getting circumcised as several had found their sexual experiences were very painful due to the skin tightening around the penis.

Personally, I am aware of several friends saying they are sorry they didn't get their sons circumcised.

COCONUT
– see Alzheimer's, cancer, Candida, Macular degeneration, Sun baking, Tooth decay, Dementia

I use coconut oil for sunbaking with a quarter of jojoba oil. As my naturopath said, "Olive oil [which I have used] bakes and coconut oil cools". Of course, I only sunbake early for about an hour and, where possible, go for a swim. Being in nature of any kind is a boost to your health and keeps up vitamin D. Bare feet absorb healing energy from the earth.

Coconuts are among the most nutritionally dense foods on the planet and have been a dietary staple for millennia. One of the reasons coconut is so special is that it's a natural food.

There is any number of articles on the internet for all the possible uses, including great for acne when rubbed in.

COD-LIVER OIL

Over many years, our family has found it great to take a teaspoon every day to relieve joint pains and swelling.

Currently I'm getting back into it for my macular-degeneration eye problem. Also, to help prevent glaucoma, which my father had.

It also helps delay bone deterioration. I've been noticing my joints click when I move, mostly in the legs, but it disappears when I religiously take the cod-liver oil. As I already take vitamin A, I only take a teaspoon of the oil. Must be careful not to take too much vitamin A as it can have side effects. It's never been a problem with me.

COLLOIDAL MINERALS

Colloidal mineral therapy was developed back in the 1930s by an Australian naturopath, Maurice Blackmore. He spent many years researching the physiological role of minerals in the process of disease and health, and he developed a system for prescribing minerals based on symptoms presented, including tongue, nail and iris signs.

The colloids differ from other minerals because they are in combinations found naturally in living tissue and are more easily absorbed by the body. Colloidal formulas consistently and quickly give good improvements.

Many of our foods lack minerals due to depleted soils, boiled food, undigested or unabsorbed food, stress and more.

Just about any kind of disorder can be caused by a lack of minerals and therefore improved by taking colloidal minerals for this reason.

These are a few of them: acne, anxiety, autistic spectrum disorders, behavioural disorders, bruising, colic, constipation, cramps, cystitis, depression, dermatitis, dry and cracked skin, eczema, fatigue, flatulence, fluid retention, gastric reflux, hair loss, headaches, indigestion, insomnia, lack of libido, menopause, menstrual irregularities, mouth ulcers, premenstrual tension, restless legs, sinuses, low sperm count, twitching muscles, weak nails and brittle hair, and so on.

The most important people who need the extra minerals are children, pregnant and lactating women, and the elderly.

COLLOIDAL SILVER

Silver has been known since ancient times to have healing and prevention of disease properties.

My aged-nursing friend from England said they used silver sheeting to wrap burn victims, and in the hospital they had many uses for it.

I find it interesting that now we can get band-aids containing silver, and my skin doctor used a patch over my sore to heal.

About 30 years ago, my naturopath suggested I buy all the silver cutlery people were throwing into the op shops as it was best to eat from them. I did buy 2 soup spoons, dessert spoons and forks, which I use. Now I'm sorry I didn't buy more.

Colloidal silver uses

Most health-food stores and pharmacies stock several brands of colloidal silver liquid and of course, you can find a vast amount of information about colloidal silver benefits on the internet.

Fascinating reading the information in a booklet I found next to a brand. The author said he had it made in Bali, and when the Bali bombing happened, he took buckets of it down to the hospital and to where the wounded were to cut the smell and stop a lot of infection.

I was so glad I had just read the leaflet one day as a young boy was screaming outside because wasps had stung him. I got him in and sprayed the area with the colloidal silver, and in a short time he was right. Never had any problems after. I had understood that the toxin can stay in your system and cause trouble for a long time.

When I was stung on my balcony by a wasp, I raced in, sprayed myself and all OK. Also, great if you do the garden watering at dusk and find you've been bitten by midges.

I have found it stops itchy skin and eyes. In fact, I use it for anything, including nasal spraying and gargling. I have been through periods of taking a teaspoonful each day as it can be helpful internally.

Now, the most effective method to get the colloidal silver into the lungs is to use a nebuliser. Generally, use one teaspoon approximately 3 times a day for 10 to 15 minutes. My nurse friend told me that doing this stopped her emphysema.

True colloidal silver doesn't contain any protein or other additives, as most of the silver content consists of nanometre-sized silver particles.

You may come across many warnings about it causing an irreversible condition called argyria (when people turn blue). However, this is caused by misuse not of true colloidal silver but of other cheaper products marketed as colloidal silver, such as ionic silver or silver protein.

One point to consider is that, because colloidal silver is such a potent antibacterial agent, you should supplement it with probiotics to ensure a proper balance of microflora.

Colloidal dosage and use

Colloidal silver (CS) needs to be applied differently for each condition. To experience colloidal silver benefits, it may be taken as follows, always keeping in mind to never use it for more than 14 days in a row:

2–5 drops applied directly to the skin

1 eyedropper taken orally for immune support

1–2 drops into eyes for pink eye

1–2 drops can help disinfect any wound or sore by applying onto a Bandaid

If prepared properly, it can be injected into a muscle, a cancerous tumour or into the bloodstream.

5 drops added into a neti pot or directly sprayed into the nose

5–10 drops can be applied vaginally or anally.

"Colloidal silver" by Margaret Hoal, (retired English nurse in her 80s, referred to above) now passed away I assume as the emails stopped 10 years ago. I never met her but she didn't have family here. She sent this to me years ago and she would be thrilled to have her cures passed on.

*To get rid of **emphysema** you need a nebuliser such as is used for asthma and other conditions as well. Pour a few ml of CS into the bowl of the nebuliser, put the mask on and switch on the machine and inhale alternately thru the nose and then the mouth for at least 5 mins. At the same time as*

inhaling, raise arms up and stretch while inhaling, leaning from one side to the other to expand further, because this expands the thorax and thus the lungs to take in more of the mist. If the ventilator she has? Buys, has a little lid or opening at the top near where the hand holding it, is, by putting a finger over that every now and again, this makes the mist finer which gets it deeper into the base of the lungs, which have to be cleaned out to get rid of the mucus.

The regimen I used is: First 2–3 days. Do this every 2 hours if possible (take a week off work!!). The next 3–4 days do it 3 hourly (but enjoy your sleep of course) and then 4 hourly for the next week or so, and once she feels she's got rid of a lot of mucus, and can take deeper breaths without coughing, and generally feels a LOT better, then do it morning and evening ongoing for a good while.

I still nebulise now and again, not because I feel that emphysema is back, but because I'm going to a cinema or something that involves being in an enclosed space and perhaps open to flu bugs, etc. And in the 7 years since I cured it, I have only had the flu once and that was 2 weeks after I had a flu injection.

I don't have those any more. I haven't even had a cold. At the same time that I had the emphysema, I also had a very noxious and persistent germ in my sputum, which had taken hold in my lungs, and the regular infections were treated with antibiotics. Do something like at least once to three times in a month, always with an antibiotic. This ceased to be funny, which is why I took the silver path. To this day, my doctor is wondering what I did to get rid of all that, but I think is too scared to ask. He knows I'm a trained nurse and nurse educator, so he has resigned himself to the fact that I do my own thing. We have a good relationship. I am blessed to have him and his understanding.

Once upon a time I had another doctor who virtually kicked me out of his practice because I consulted a naturopath which made me better, and I thought he would be pleased!!

The only thing I haven't had done since the cure, is have another lung function test to "prove" the emphysema is gone. This is because I no longer have any symptoms of emphysema, so the test is not justified.

I am not a doctor, and I am simply telling you what I did, and the results of that. Colloidal silver was used during the First World War and even in the Second World War to treat infected wounds, as until 1940 something, there was no penicillin

Even in the '60s, we were treating burned children by wrapping them up in sheets soaked in silver nitrate to prevent infection. In the olden days people used to keep milk fresher by putting a silver coin in the bottle. Also keeping water fresh.

That old furphy of turning blue can only happen (as it did with the "blue bloods" of European royalty) when the silver being imbibed is not colloidal, viz., it's like 'raw' (particle) silver. They ate and drank out of silver goblets and platters. The acidity of the wine and some foods dissolved the metal silver so to speak, and that's why they were blueish.

To be colloidal (as opposed to particle) silver, requires a "generator" that dissolves the silver off the pure silver elements used with the generator in distilled water (and not just any old type. It has to be a good type) That dissolving process causes the dissolved silver to be IONIC rather than PARTICLE.

When you take CS by mouth which you should do alongside the nebulising, take about 20 to 30 ml, 2 to 3 times a day. The best distribution of the silver through the body is via the nebuliser, but for any gastro-enteric, urinary-tract, etc. infections, by mouth is a must AS WELL AS the nebuliser.

How does it work, you may ask? The silver in the fine ionic solution gets between the bacteria/virus and its food source. The cell, so the bacteria/virus is starved. CS works wonders on cold/flu using the nasal spray plus the nebuliser, and by mouth, for everything as well.

Kits for making colloidal silver are available to make your own. I love my kit.

COLOUR and LIGHT

– see Black, Yellow

Colour is now known to influence healing as does music.

We can be exposed to colours, light ribbons and any other sorts of colour, even psychically to help stimulate health to the damaged area.

People notice certain colours can also stimulate emotions. Everyone who walks past my very yellow painting of sunflowers comments, "It makes me feel happy".

Red

It was found that when participants at a conference were put in a room with red light, they had a higher level of brain activity associated with alertness, stimulated and they felt more energy. My acupuncture man told me to stay off spiced red food and stay with the cooler flavours and colours as my blood was too hot. Dark red is also the first chakra related to sexual action.

Orange

Orange foods such as sweet potato, carrots and pumpkin get their colour from carotenoids like beta-carotene, which may play an important role in reproduction and progesterone. In chakras, orange is the second one and is about the area of good social stimulation.

Yellow

Yellow is a curious colour. It seems to be the colour that most people are drawn to, and the one that is most correlated with a normal mood. It is of course the colour of the sun which is important for healing. It is also good for mental stimulation so not so good for a bedroom.

Green

Researchers have discovered some fascinating links associating the colour green with the heart. It is the colour related to money (green-back dollar) new growth, Spring. People feel cool in a green room or in a forest. This can include cooling the heart. It is opposite to red in the colour spectrum.

Blue

The colour blue has powerful effects on the brain and memory. Not so good if you want to sleep as people can be wanting to complete tasks during the night.

It has been shown that people performed better on a working memory task and had greater activation in the prefrontal regions of the brain after being in a blue light.

Blue and shades of it are the top chakras so not surprising it stimulates the brain.

White

Bright light has been found to be helpful in non-seasonal depression.

Doctors and nutritionists have been saying for some time, "Eat lots of fruit and vegetables in a variety of colours for good health".

Red: pomegranate, strawberry, beet
Orange: apricot, carrot, orange
Yellow: lemon, pineappl
Green: broccoli, kale, mint
Blue: blueberry, bilberry
White: coconut, banana, cauliflower

Artificial light and health

Artificial light has made a great change in our lives since it was invented.   There are many forms and has made a big difference to work areas as well as homes. This means that it is radiating light and colour into the space which can and does affect people working there and can have side affects.

I have found that my 2 friends with melanoma in their 80s have almost never been in the sun and rarely in their childhood. Many other sun-mad friends haven't had any problems. I've often wondered if it is something in the lighting at home or office, television, etc. all emitting light that could be affecting them.

A doctor who had erratic periods decided to leave the light on for a few days in the middle of the month and found that it kept her periods in cycle. Obviously he right kind of light.

Another interesting fact was women had menstrual troubles under pink fluorescents light but okay under the blue ones. Keeping a hat on when working under fluorescent lighting stops the lights above from affecting you.

We are now warned that there is a light emitted from our computer screens which is damaging the eyes. I now have the special glasses to protect me.

Colours and Astrology

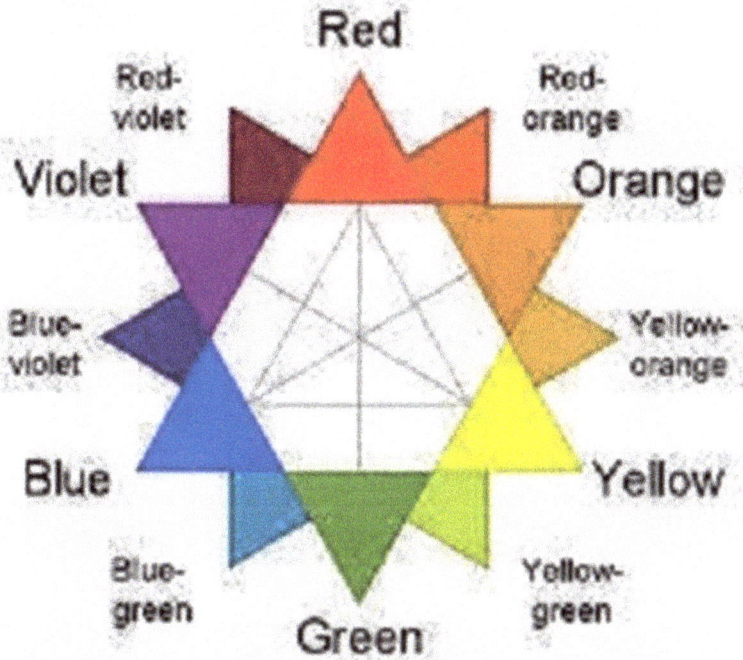

There are 2 powers that work in the world: one is colour and the other is vibration. Every person and thing, even words and feelings, have colours. The planet and astrology work according to these colours.

Colours have been given to the planets and astrology signs as well as the chakras.

D

DEATH, DYING, GRIEF and AFTERLIFE

This is a huge topic so I will give you the name of a few books that will be very helpful to read. One fascinating article I read years ago was about how in a ward in the UK they decided to weigh a person before death and then after. They did this several times and found that exactly the same loss of weight happened to everyone. I think it was about ¼ kilo, though not sure exactly. What could that be? The spirit or what?

Elisabeth Kubler-Ross first brought into the public awareness in the western world in her book, **On Death and Dying**. Other religions and cultures have included this subject in their everyday life, whereas there is so much fear about death in the Western world.

Several books I read many years ago really help drop any fear I had of dying. They are:

Love, Medicine & Miracles by Bernie Siegel.

A Way to Die: Living until the end by Rosemary and Victor Zorza. This is the story of Jane Zorza.

Two inspiring recent books are:

Dying to be Me: My journey from cancer, to near death, to true healing by Anita Moorjani.

Proof of Heaven: A neurosurgeon's journey into the afterlife by Eben Alexander.

Coping with grief by Mal and Dianne McKissock. We used this little book in counselling.

It is important for people to take time to grieve and not feel guilty because they are angry or dwelling on what they could have done to help. When a person isn't recovering, they may need professional help.

Postcards from the Other Side: True stories from the afterlife by Michelle and Ezio de Angelis.

DEMENTIA

– see Alzheimer's

How to tell the difference between dementia and normal aging

As more brain researchers are finding that subjective cognitive complaints may be the earliest sign of Alzheimer's disease, how can you tell the difference between normal age-related memory problems and early Alzheimer's? The following 10 warning signs from the Alzheimer's Association will help you differentiate between the two:

1. significant memory changes
2. difficulty solving problems or making plans
3. difficulty completing familiar tasks at home, work and play
4. confusion with time or place
5. trouble understanding visual images and spatial relationships
6. new problems with words in speaking or writing
7. misplacing things and losing the ability to retrace steps
8. decreased or poor judgement
9. withdrawal from work or social activities
10. changes in mood and personality.

Adhering to a balanced Mediterranean style diet is associated with slower cognitive decline. This is recommended for good health. Having vitamins D and B9 can also help.

Some people are getting good results from adding coconut oil. Sage and Rosemary teas are also good for short-term memory. I certainly have found them helpful.

DENTAL

– see Teeth

Dental root canal therapy – A high percentage of cancer patients have had root canal.

During a root canal, there is no way to sterilise your tooth, afterwards, dangerous bacteria hide out in the tooth and are unreachable with antibiotics.

Root-canalled and filled teeth harbour bacteria that morph into very toxic forms, which then can migrate to other tissues in your body and cause serious medical conditions, including diseases of your heart, kidneys, bones, and brain.

There is no other medical practice that permits leaving a dead body part inside your body, because it triggers your immune system to attack.

If you have a diseased tooth, or if you've already had a root canal, it is recommended consulting a biological dentist about having it extracted. Have to say I've kept mine but refuse any more so end up getting the tooth out.

Each tooth in acupuncture has a meridian to an organ, which means infection, damage and so on will affect the organ or vice versa.

When people have the tooth out, the organ can heal. One woman with a lot of health problems had to have her teeth out for some reason or other, and her health improved considerably.

I know that health retreats, where people with cancer go to hopefully heal, ask patients to get their teeth cleared for mercury and generally checked out before they will give treatment.

DEPRESSION
– see Black, Death and Dying

There have been several times in my life when I've been depressed during childhood, in my marriage and for 5 years after that. Also, during much of my years of personal growth in my 40s, I wouldn't take drugs to help, though later in my 50s, when I did my Diploma in Psychotherapy and Relationship Counselling, I came to understand it can be helpful to get relief medically while having counselling.

There are many causes for depression and many ways of healing. Personally, after years of depression, it helped when (while doing personal-growth group) I stopped myself from thinking about what could have been and what I could have had, what I didn't have and what I wanted. Be in the NOW.

Instead, I learned to accept what I had (gratitude) and where I was at. Then decide what to do NOW. Also, life is about 10% what happens to you and 90% how you handle it. Take some kind of action regarding my situation instead of feeling a victim, I changed the subject so to speak, and it brought improvement slowly but surely.

Another great help was finding out about what was happening in my astrological chart, which indicated that certain planets were helping create stress and that it wouldn't last forever. When depressed, we always think it will go on forever. Saturn is generally regarded as the planet most related to depression.

Given a timeline for the planets to move, I found it easier to work on the situations that were being affected: For example, father/partner issues, lack of work/education and health knowing it would be resolved to some degree soon.

Counselling and therapy can do wonders, especially when combined with group therapy. We realise that we are not the only ones in misery and sometimes someone else seems worse off (or we can help them). Then we can feel that maybe things aren't too bad with us.

If people prefer to use the standard drugs, they need to use them in combination with counselling/therapy and some homeopathy, more healthy food, etc. Then gradually cut down on drugs/alcohol, which usually act as a depressant, as you feel better.

St John's Wort is often suggested by naturopaths, and there are many other homeopathic, herbal treatments and teas that can be used.

DIABETICS

– see Sugar – Weight

Too much sugar and foods that create sugar are the main causes for diabetes and weight. Of course, many of us have emotional issues related to taking so much sugar.

These days it is common for women to get a form of diabetes when pregnant, along with putting on a lot of weight.

Years ago, we weren't allowed to put on weight. The weight was checked by the doctor consistently when we went for the check-ups. Near the end, I remember mine saying that if I put on more weight, he would send me to hospital. So I revised my intake of food and had great results.

DIET

– see Fat, Diabetics

Weight loss and reduced breathing

Ever wonder why it is so difficult if not impossible, to lose weight when you are eating practically nothing? Many people go on intensive diets and do lose weight only to see the pounds come back the moment they end their diet. This is more than frustrating! Everyone comes out with a different diet that has fantastic promises but there is something that is not being addressed that is important to everyone – not just overweight people.

Our weight can be hereditary, in how we feel about ourselves, to what we eat, to our insulin sensitivity, to the amount of exercise we get, and so on. Also, many think they are hungry when in fact they are thirsty.

I met someone recently who said he lost 16 kg by stopping sugar and processed food. I was impressed.

Many are finding it isn't necessary to go on strict diets but to eat differently with much smaller servings. Recognised they were eating as if they were still growing or as they did in their younger years and weren't doing much exercise.

Eating lots more fruit (it gives fibre and natural sugar which the body needs) and vegetables helps lift the acidity that comes about when not eating, processing, or breathing properly.

Yoga and regular exercise are essential. Most people find these the hardest to do as it means taking time out for themselves from their busy days.

Work out a physical activity you might enjoy. Dancing is very good. Maybe do yoga or exercise class one day and dance one night. Sharing the exercise makes it easier, and once you are feeling fitter or more able to play with children the happier you feel.

When I was in a personal-growth group, several people started to lose weight and one girl realised she couldn't get her wedding dress made until almost on the day, as she was losing so much weight due to her psychological release and attitude.

One of the men at 35 was a virgin living at home, a good Catholic boy. As he moved along, he started to gain some self-worth, dressing better, moved out of home and started dating. His weight dropped considerably.

It was all through realising how they saw themselves and what they'd come to expect along with unknown fear. Once they were facing and resolving these issues weight dropped away. Much to everyone's surprise.

DISEASE

DIS – EASE

Questions you need to ask when not well:

What am I learning about myself by having this disease?

What is this disease?

What is this condition?

What is this situation forcing me to face?

What issues have come up because of this disease that may not have come up if I didn't have it?

How does it serve me to have this disease?

What am I learning by creating it?

Read *Love your Disease: It's Keeping you Healthy* by John Harrison.

My notes at a Nexus conference 2014 talk called "Disease" by Don Chisholm
(These are rough notes but you can follow up with details on his web site.)

Our bodies contain 99% molecules of water. Our bacteria cells are non-human and we need them, both good and bad. There are 500 species.

Poor absorption causes illness. Generally, children are on worse diets since the Second World War.

Cancer used to be random in the '70s, but by 2040 we will all get cancer, according to statistics.

Ninety-eight per cent of people with cancer have had root canal therapy leaving dead teeth in our head.

In the '70s, autism was 1 in 10,000. In 2013 it was 1 in 50. In 2014, it was 1 in 7.

Aspartame is in much of our food and it is not meant to be heated.

Ninety-three per cent of experts say genetically modified food (GM) is not good for us. Weed killer is now in soy and in syrups and most manufactured food.

One hundred and fifty thousand farmers in India have committed suicide because they can't feed their family. Once they saved seed from crops and planted them the next year, but GM is dead and they must buy seeds every year which they can't afford.

Parasites are always in us with cancer. With oxygen there is no cancer. Candida gives us the sugar craving and most of the food we love is desired by the Candida (sugar added to everything).

Scientist work on making fake smell, flavour, colour to food to tempt us to buy. In the taste of strawberry, there are 3,500 chemicals and the little things that look like seeds can be tiny bits of wood.

Up to 1930, there was virtually no disease except tuberculosis, (TB) and sexual diseases. People died from accidents, childbirth, starvation, and drowning.

DNA

Many people want to know through DNA what their health risks are, and even in astrology they can note weaknesses and patterns in families which appear to cause a certain health problem.

A book written by Bruce H. Lipton is **The Biology of Belief: Unleashing the power of consciousness matter & miracles** is really worth reading. Lipton, who was at the forefront of DNA research, brings up the fact that in the end the environment that people are exposed to, both physical and emotional, will usually outweigh the DNA. This means that if we don't follow in family footsteps of food, beliefs, etc. we don't get the family health problems.

We differentiate, doing our own thing and not relying on family or community for acceptance or approval.

Also, as members of the Fellowship of First Fleeters, we are finding people are doing DNA tests to prove who they are and can join. However, it is more complicated than that. We must know the history as well as check the DNA. Luckily, we have a couple of expert members on the subject to help.

If birth certificates can be changed in future due to lesbian, gay, bisexual and transgender (LGBT), it will be hard to trace families. Hard enough when people use the wife's surname for the children, which happens for various reasons.

E

EAR – HEARING
– see Face and Hair

The external ear has the ends of all the meridians in it round the rim which is why acupuncture can be helpful here for some health problems as well as on the body. It was used a lot for weight a while ago. Haven't heard of it lately.

Earaches are caused by many things: like not wanting to hear what is going on in the home. I had dreadful earaches as a child, so I really believe in that. Add my crossed eye not wanting to see what was going on or how to stop it. Also, there are things children push in there, bugs getting in and so on.

Tipping in a little warm olive oil into your ear can help, or a teaspoon of peroxide can kill infections. I would also use colloidal silver (see information under C) in the ear to kill bacteria. In recent years, I found ear candling very good for clearing the wax in my ears.

It has been noted in the book, **Sound therapy: Music to Recharge your Brain** by Patricia and Rafaele Joudry, that the ear can turn off listening early in life if a child doesn't want to hear things (autism, poor hearing).

Hearing, reading, stress, tinnitus and many more problems can be healed. Classical music is so much better for hearing and healing than the heavy, loud banging rock. It was found that a 25-year old's hearing can be as bad as that of a 50-year-old man in a factory.

EARTHQUAKE

For my readers living in earthquake areas and the many who travel overseas to such areas, you may find this helpful.

I saw on television an Australian girl saying she had no idea what to do when she was caught overseas in an earthquake. Rang her mother who of course had no idea, so stood under a door frame as she thought she'd heard to do. Actually, it is not.

These tips could be of help

Ducking for cover under a door frame or desk, you will likely get crushed as they move away in one direction or the other.

Animals and babies naturally curl up in foetal position, and so should we. It makes a smaller space. Also curl up next to an object like the sofa but leave a space next to it.

Wooden buildings are a safer type of building to be in. Wood is flexible and moves with the force of the earthquake. If it collapses, large survival voids are created, and wood doesn't have the weight of other materials.

If in bed, roll off to the floor (not under) as a rough void will exist around the bed.

Don't go to the stairs as they have a different speed and swing separately and keep moving longer, caused by banging into each other. They can still crash later with people on them, etc.

Stay near the outer walls or outside them. It will be less likely that the escape route is blocked.

Staying inside the car allows for things to crash on you. Best to get out and sit or lie next to them as there will be a void around it even if crushed by concrete.

Large voids are made around stacks of paper in the office as it doesn't compact.

EARTHING

In recent years, some podiatrists and natural therapists have come to realise our lack of connecting physically to the earth is not good for our health. We are always much healthier when we spend time on the beach in bare feet, walking barefooted, gardening, etc.

In Japan, some doctors recommend going into the forest to absorb nature for better health.

We used to have leather or wooden shoes and houses built on wood and bamboo. Today we live in a synthetic, plastic world for much of the time. Decking and floorboards absorb the earth energy so are therefore good to sit on.

Plastic shoes, houses built on concrete with plastic sheeting is the norm. This means we lack the natural-healing earth energy that is good for us.

There are many products made now that you can use in the house if you can't get out to walk barefooted. Most of my childhood was in bare feet, through winter and summer. We refused to wear shoes where possible. Check the internet for more information on earthing.

EGGS

– see Osteoporosis – Bones, Burns

Eggs can have many uses. The white can be good for some things and the yolk for others. Eggs are high in protein. However, too many eggs can be bad for the liver. Great to eat every morning.

My sister was born with jaundice and small thyroid lump. Our naturopath took her off eggs and cheese, the liver may cause jaundice. She eventually came to eat them but has never been that keen on them.

At one stage we had egg yolk beaten up in orange juice before breakfast (naturopath's suggestion), as it was very good for us. Loved it. We had lots of meringues or pavlova to use up the white. This was handy for my mother being a minister's wife who needed such things for morning and afternoon teas/meetings with parishioner groups.

The shell can be used for bone development – see Osteoporosis

EMF

– see Cancer, Mobiles, Radiation, Sleep, Wireless, WiFi

Radios, braces, earrings, hip replacements and metal can increase wireless radiation and absorption into the body (also underwire bras).

Published research indicates that metal implants affect electromagnetic radiation absorption in the body.

Some say that metal earrings, watches and metal glasses also attract more EMF.

People have a variety of metal implants in their body from dental implants, the pins used for broken bones, hip replacements and brain implants. Metallic implants inside the body have become a serious concern that regulatory agencies have not addressed.

Experts say when pregnant keep clear where possible of electronics near their body, and that includes standing by a microwave under the bench when changing a nappy

EMF from mobiles

EMF is an invisible zone of energy that surrounds electric devices, and wiring is very unhealthy for you.

EMFs comprise 2 fields: an electric field and a magnetic field.

The electric field is created by voltage, which determines the force. Most electric fields can be shielded by the design of the appliance, or physically, by walls or other barriers.

The magnetic field is created by the current, which is the amount of electricity being pushed. This is the main cause of health concerns as it can travel through most barriers for long distances and is difficult to block.

There have been many scientists, medical experts, etc. who have advised against it but are ignored. So many laws about it are 20 years old and not updated to the current devices.

It concludes that the existing standards for public safety are completely inadequate to protect your health. There is evidence that electromagnetic fields have shown it can cause many diseases and health problems including DNA

A famous New South Wales brain surgeon was on television the other day saying brain cancer and similar have had a dramatic rise in recent years particularly among young people which maybe a cause.

It is said that the iPhone, Apple's smartphone, comes with the advice that you should keep your phone at least 15 mm away from your body at all times. This may come as a surprise to those who always keep the phone in their pockets.

When I see people with their mobiles attached to their belt or in their back pocket with the top of the aerial pointing to the kidneys, they can expect some health issues in that area over time. One man found once he stopped putting the phone in his chest pocket then his heart problems cleared. Luckily it hadn't been too damaged at that stage.

There are guides which come with all phones suggesting it not be near the body but rarely does anyone read them, including me. Seems so hard to understand. For example, the BlackBerry guide suggests that users, particularly pregnant women and teenagers, keep their phone 25 mm from their body. It is in the car as well now.

Sometimes when feeling a bit wonky in the car, I wonder is it the Bluetooth affecting me.

Some years ago, instead of my phone, I talked on a hands-free phone near the bed (now know it has more radiation than a mobile) for 3 hours and afterwards I thought my head would explode. Can't explain the terrible feeling but I've never talked for more than a few minutes on a hands-free phone since, except when absolutely necessary. That doesn't happen on a landline, which I cling to for several good reasons.

Recently I lost my mobile which was on aeroplane mode due to being in a meeting. I went home but there were no neighbours around. Luckily, I had a landline (probably not for long) and a computer on my desk, so I was able to ring around people (I keep their numbers in an address book as well as on the phone) and I was advised to look up the internet and put in "Where's my phone" which enabled me to find it.

I have found the landline rescued me in another similar situation, so I am all for it, though most family and friends now only have mobile though many of them wish they had their landline as well. I would have been completely stumped if I didn't have the landline.

Radiofrequency radiation (RF) and public health policy

Though it is not advertised, governments around the world are questioning the use of electronics in schools. Many are banning it in schools or in certain areas as they have found it has a bad effect on children and their behaviour. Of course, teachers with headaches and health problems not noticed previously.

Now at least schools are beginning to ban mobiles for the bad effect it has on concentration, social contact, possible brain cancer and learning.

Children are also becoming addicted, which is affecting the brain and ability to concentrate for more than a short time.

There are now many items being made to deflect the electromagnetic field (EMF) and to protect against the radiation such as disks to put on your phone, in the car, on the computer and on the body. I have a plug that goes into the electrical system at home to counteract it in the house.

EMPHYSEMA

– "Colloidal silver" by Margaret Hoal, Eyes, Vegetables

EPSOM SALTS

– see Magnesium

It is a natural remedy for many health conditions. Epsom salt can also relax the nervous system and soothe the body, mind, and soul.

The magnesium content in Epsom salt is particularly valuable. It aids in calcium absorption and plays a key role in the formation of bones and teeth. It also plays an important role in maintaining cardiovascular health by stabilising heart rhythm, preventing abnormal blood clotting and supporting normal blood pressure levels.

These salts can be used in many ways to clear toxins and smooth skin. You can add some essential oils as well to the bath.

Great to throw half a pack in the bath to clear acidity and infections. Use with cold water for sunburn, bug bites, sore muscles, soak feet in for pedicure, massage into wet skin after shower, then rinse off.

ESSENTIAL OILS

– see Cancer

I won't go through all the oils – only a few that I have been interested in. They are used for emotional support and healing. My favourite aromas around the house are pine, peppermint, orange, marjoram, myrrh and bergamot.

I was going down with a cold when travelling for work years ago. So I decided to use the oils I had with me – peppermint, bergamot and eucalyptus – in a bowl of hot water and put my face over it with a towel over me. Certainly was a big help.

Frankincense – Also known as Boswellia, tests are showing it may be a safe and effective remedy for women who suffer from ovarian cancer and of course much more.

Lavender and marjoram – These 2 essential oils are known as the most relaxing of the essential oils and used to help sleep. Put drops on your pillow, on your skin and a tissue to rest on your chest. Also, deep breathe them in when turning out the lights.

Lavender is also good for clearing smells. Spray it on the item or dab it on. **Coffee** is also good for absorbing smells.

Myrrh – I love this to use on mouth ulcers and infections in the mouth. I must admit, I use it straight rather than with water on the spot, and it is usually gone within a day or so.

A few drops in your face cream does wonders for the skin.

As a friend was having problems with inflammation and problems with his anus, I suggested to him that if myrrh works to heal in a wet mouth, then it might be very helpful for him. Forgot to check later how it went but worth a try.

Eucalyptus oil – The most commonly used eucalyptus varieties traditionally been Eucalyptus globulus and Eucalyptus radiata for aromatherapy and general purposes. But science is discovering that dozens of other varieties of eucalyptus have excellent healing qualities as well.

Ancient aboriginal uses of eucalyptus

Australian aboriginal people have a history dating back tens of thousands of years and they used eucalyptus extensively for healing. They bound the leaves around serious wounds to prevent infection and promote healing. They knew the fresh, lung-opening aroma to be excellent for clearing respiratory congestion, and that it helped to suppress coughing.

They used eucalyptus to repel the ever-present outback flies and insects, and employed eucalyptus as a rub for sore muscles, joint pain, and headaches.

Sometimes they would burn the leaves and inhale the smoke to relieve a fever. Even the resin of the eucalyptus tree was collected, boiled, and used as a disinfectant for treating cuts, sores, and other painful conditions. Other cultures use eucalyptus as well. For instance, traditional Chinese and Indian (Ayurvedic) medicine employed the use of eucalyptus for a wide range of medical conditions.

How eucalyptus essential oil was brought to the West

In 1848, Joseph Bosisto, a young pharmacist from Yorkshire, England, arrived in Australia thinking he was going to take part in the Victorian gold rush. Instead, he began to investigate the healing properties of Australian plants, specifically eucalyptus. In 1852, he began distilling eucalyptus oil, making it one of the oldest commercially available oils. Eucalyptus oil became a highly sought-after medicinal oil, it even won prizes in 17 international exhibitions in 1891!

Eucalyptus was used extensively during both world wars. It was used to control meningitis and influenza outbreaks, and to cleanse wounds when other antibacterial supplies ran out. In the 1940s and '50s, many cold-and-cough medicines contained eucalyptus oil for it was widely known then for its ability to ease those conditions.

IN THE HOUSE It is very good to rub into labels that are stuck onto furniture or glass. This is the best way to lift/scrub them off with no damage to the furniture.

Great to use in the washing machine if a lot of oily towels, etc. need washing.

EYES

– see Introduction, Iridology, Face and Hair, Iridology, Coconut, Heart, Macular (front of the book)

There is a famous saying, something like "Eyes are the window to the soul". They are certainly registering all your internal health. Iridology is a brilliant way to get a diagnosis of what's wrong. I get my eyes checked every year. Several times people find that something is forming in the body long before the symptoms show.

I had a turned eye as a child, which was healed naturally with exercises and a patch over the good eye to strengthen the turned eye. A total misery at school with teasing me over my patch I wore for years. However, in my 50's, my eye started to slide again and ended up getting the operation when I was 62. Seems there was no pension, etc. discount because a paediatric doctor does it. I asked him if he did many adults. He said that he still did a few.

An excellent way to heal eyes and clear the acidity is by using an eye bath and clearing the acidity every day. Use filtered clean water (fluoride is shown not to be good for eyes). The water can sting, which means they need cleaning. Roll the eyes sideways, up and down and round and round. At the end of a session, there should be no stinging. This can also be done when swimming in salt water.

Glasses can weaken your eyes so now I only use them for reading and driving. Have to say I'm a bit lazy on eye fitness and find them sliding again now nearly 20 years on. However, I'm doing some exercising but also have connected with healers who explain my brain needs clearing along with acupuncture in that area, and I need to add affirmations with the exercises. My eyes are quite improved.

There are several organisations which do healing eyesight. I know a man who no longer wears glasses after doing a course. One way of improving eyesight is to not use tinted glasses or sunglasses, which I decided to work on, and don't wear them anymore. I trained myself by wearing a hat with a brim, which cuts the glare. I also dropped the sun visor in the car.

It also helps to read outdoors without the glasses if possible. You will notice that black and white is much easier to read than when they use colour on colour, etc. It is the contrast which helps the eyes.

As a child, and sometimes even now, I had to deal with **styes** (what didn't I want to look at?) Once I had to stay home from school with 7 on one eye and 4 on another. It was so painful to open and close my eyes. (It seems I didn't want to see the anger and disruption in the family.)

Apart from the eye cleaning, I used Golden Eye ointment. For years as an adult, I have used a good gold ring (don't think my family had any gold in my childhood). I rub it on the area and it clears up. May have to rub many times a day, and firmly, so it breaks up.

Another help with itching and styes is colloidal silver. Spray it in and on your eyes and it seems to clear very quickly Itchy eyes are related to the liver.

Something in your eye? Use the heel of your hand and bang it on your head just above the eye, slightly to the side. I know it looks funny when you're in the street. However, it really works to clear your eye before you rub it and wreck your make up. If it's an eyelash in the eye, it may not work as it sticks to the eye.

Lutein is a naturally occurring carotenoid and is used by your body as a powerful antioxidant, and by your eyes for blue-light absorption, able to fight free radicals and protect cells from oxidative damage.

Lutein is found in green leafy vegetables like spinach and kale, also in carrots, squash, and other orange and yellow fruits, vegetables, and eggs.

The highest concentration of lutein in your eye is in your macula – the tiny central part of your retina responsible for straight-ahead and detailed vision. More specifically, lutein is found in the macular pigment – known for helping to protect your central vision.

Improve eyesight – My notes on a talk by Janet Goodridge at Noosa Library. (Her mother developed this first in Australia.)

They have developed a set of exercises using a CD and pinhole glasses which corrects eyesight. Janet runs regular workshops.

Myopia – short sighted – I don't know what these mean but an optometrist would.

1.30	1.75	180
3.75	2.00	75

Turned eye more tricky

Long sighted + sphere

There are 7 muscles in the eye – 6 large exterior and 1 interior.

They move in shape pairs.

If the skull bone is compressed where a set is attached, it can cause turned eye.

Need antioxidant – lots of vitamin C, fruit. Vitamin A for night vision – sunlight helps.

Personality types related to these eye problems

Myopia – shy people, perfectionist, concerned what others think, worrier, etc. It switches the R brain to L. Outer vision is blurry. There is stress, unresolved fear. They make good accountants.

Presbyopia – not such stress. I'm too busy to take time for myself.

Hyperopia – glasses for reading, great long-distance sight. Hate sitting still, rather be out there. Difficult, tantrums, temper. The artist, muso, designer, etc. Unresolved anger. R brain activated.

Astigmatism – Most changeable. Eyesight different at different times of day and have different prescriptions. TRAUMA can be from something as simple as move of house, parents not available, so not safe to change. Need to clear the pain and anger and review prescription to improve sight. Sensitive, defensive people.

Saccadic motion – Enables eyesight.

The more light you get into your eyes, the better sight you get. Exercises help get more in.

Sunglasses are addictive. The more you wear them, the more you need them but they cut the light and especially bad for night vision. Best to use a wide-brim hat, etc. to cut the glare.

Sadly, I have got all the information and prepared myself to do the healing course at home years ago (I'm not good at home learning) but realise I work better in workshops and just never got to take the time each day to work on it. Hope to do it one day at a workshop.

My father suffered from glaucoma and my mother macular degeneration. This means I usually have my eyes tested at least every 2 years. In fact, people with any of these issues in their families need to have regular eye check-ups even if they don't notice any eye problems. Also, their siblings, children and grandchildren should be checked because when the symptoms show it can be too late and a lot harder to deal with.

My eyesight is so important to me due to my love of colour, photography and painting, so I donate to most of the organisations.

F

FACE and HAIR

In Chinese medicine, they say the face shows our health.

Mouth and chin

Smoking and certain things like pursing your lips and frowning create wrinkles. When you find some wrinkles are forming, I suggest you take note of what you are thinking or doing related to them and make an effort to stop doing it or let go of the worry.

Help your face to relax by doing face exercise, like closing your mouth and gently blowing out of your mouth while closed – it puffs out the lips. Stretch your neck by pulling your head back and forward. Gently lift up your face from the mouth and around your eyes. I use some olive oil or face cream while doing this.

Sores around the mouth can indicate lack of vitamin B so step up your intake of food with vitamin B or get supplement pills.

Dry lips: this can help you realise you are not drinking enough water and need vitamins to dry skin.

Dry skin/inflammation on the chin: can be related to digestion and bowels

Ears and jawline

Itchy ears could be allergy. Psoriasis and eczema are signs that the person is depleted in vitamin D – the sunshine vitamin – and is irritable. Spending 10 minutes with face (eyes closed) exposed to the sun is healing.

Acne on the jawline: Refined food, sugar, burgers and chips and fizzy drinks can cause acne. Often teens are into this kind of food, especially if not eating properly at home. Try eating apricots, sweet potato and any similar coloured food to give more vitamin A.

Eyes

It is good to release the toxins in the eyes by exposing them closed to the sun for about 10 minutes.

If dark circles under the eyes persist despite regular and restful sleep this may be a result of intolerance to diary food. Sufferers should remove dairy and wheat along with too much alcohol.

Forehead

Horizontal lines on the forehead: can be digestive issues. So drinking warm water with lemon juice every morning can help. I also have a spoon of anti-inflammatory turmeric powder in mine.

A pronounced frown line between the eyes can indicate liver problems which of course can be brought about by many things. Not just alcohol and poor food. This could be for physical, environmental and emotional reasons also, which eventually leads to affecting the other organs and causes burnout.

Skin

Spots on the cheeks show the skin could be a bit clogged up. Go without makeup for periods of time to allow the skin to breathe. Go free in the house. I use aloe vera at least once a week. When dry, cover with coconut or olive oil.

I think far too many women have facials, which take away the natural oils. Some skins are already too dry, others just right, but want to make sure it is clean so get the facials. The few times I had a facial, it just somehow felt too dry and smooth (sort of plastic feel), though they put any number of creams, etc. on.

Oily skin can be caused by diet and/or not the right skin creams/makeup. Dry skin can do with more oily foods because our body becomes more dehydrated as we get older.

Lots of water (room temperature) helps cleanse the system

About 20 years ago, I read that almost all shampoo, skin products, house cleansers, sunscreen, washing powders have a lot of chemicals in them which can cause cancer used over a period of time. Individually they may be considered to contain the safe amount but when you add the products together then it is far too much.

I started checking labels to avoid the most cancer forming toxic chemicals of paraben, solidum lauryl sulphate, formaldehyde, DEA, TEA, PEG and propylene glycol and it was very hard to find anything free of them and if free, very expensive. Though I noted one of the supposedly most healthy ranges has some of these chemicals in them.

Now there are a lot of these products available for the skin that are free of the chemicals.

In checking this I was also shocked to see the long line of chemicals in cakes (which I rarely buy) at the supermarket. At home, it might take something like 6 ingredients rather than 15 or more. This is the same with ice cream, not much in milk.

Elsewhere on your head

Sore throats and ulcers can be a sign of a gum infection. Mouth ulcers can indicate a suppressed immune system, so rest and eat well. I use a few dabs of myrrh on them. For my throat, I gargle with apple cider vinegar or colloidal silver and use propolis liquid sprayed in the back of the throat to kill infection. Sipping a mix of equal lemon and olive oil feels great also.

Bad breath means you need to check liver and diet along with a dental check-up.

Dry mouth can be a sign of diabetes or just dehydration.

Yellow teeth usually means too much tea. Also, coffee and smoking can cause discoloured teeth.

Dull, brittle hair can mean you are low in protein. A diet rich in iron and essential fatty acids will also help keep it strong. Rapid thinning can be thyroid.

The spiritual nature of hair – Deva Kaur Khalsa, yoga teacher

She says our hair has all kinds of value apart from decorative. Vitality being part of it.

We are the only creature who grows longer hair on our head as we grow into adulthood. Left uncut, your hair will grow to a particular length and then stop all by itself at the correct length for you.

Many believe that people who have long hair tend to be less tired, more energetic and less likely to become depressed. People who have long hair also conserve energy and don't feel the cold of winter the same as people with short hair.

Think of the story of Samson and Delilah in the Bible! He lost his strength when she cut his hair. Another example of the power of hair was when they humiliated the conquered people of China. Genghis Khan made them cut their hair and wear bangs over the forehead! (Bangs/fringes cover the 3rd eye, inhibiting intuition and subtle knowledge.)

Also, when the Europeans arrived in China, they got rid of the men's pigtails. Later on the communists didn't allow long hair.

Hair is an extension of the nervous system

Something never mentioned during Vietnam war, and discovered by a psychologist working in the early nineties at a Veterans Affairs medical hospital, was an experiment done related to hair.

He worked with combat veterans with post-traumatic stress disorder (PTSD). Most of them had served in Vietnam. The psychologist was shocked to read about a special Indian team and the effect that cutting their hair had on them.

The veterans were supposed to be good at knowing when people were moving towards them from a great distance, which would be a great help for the army. Traditionally they slept on the floor and had long hair. However, once all were dressed in army uniform, haircut and tested, they discovered it didn't work. I found this fascinating.

Interesting that in the '60s longer hair was worn by most people and really long hair (mostly hippies) was the norm. Turned out to be a very creative time, and people looked for the spiritual side of life.

FASTING

– see Grapes

Fasting for as little as 3 days can regenerate the entire immune system, even in the elderly, scientists have found in a breakthrough. My Chinese medicine man says it isn't always good as some people aren't nourished enough already. Need to be sure it won't have a poor effect.

Though fasting can be like a regeneration switch (like when we turn the computer off to restart), getting the immune system and the white blood cells a restart.

It is wise to check with your naturopath, etc. if there is a reason that you should or shouldn't fast. In some situations, it would not be wise to do so, such as being pregnant.

My healer says that I don't seem to get enough nourishment from my food and my ying and yang are so erratic that I shouldn't fast. Maybe only for a day.

Although using the grape diet keeps me nourished at the same time as clearing things out. Written about in section Fruit and then read Grapes.

FAT

– see Arthritis, Cancer, Diabetes, Premenstrual syndrome (PMS)

There wasn't the obesity back years ago when people ate quite a bit of natural fat made at home from the meat. We used to love dripping on our bread. So many doctors and manufacturers over the last 50 years have told us that it is bad for you and can cause heart trouble, cholesterol and weight gain, (I don't think they were much of a problem before).

Why would they say that? Because natural fat is not owned by manufacturers, patented, or trademarked. They could corner the market and sell it to you at a huge profit.

So they have created all sorts of fat substitutes to use instead of the real thing

Fat in nature and have a fixed cost. But carbohydrates that they have pushed can be grown in huge quantities: get the government to subsidise and pay you for growing them, and sell them for cheaper than dirt.

You need this nutrient of fat to give you energy, maintain your body temperature, transport nutrients, and build a faster brain. Fat is so important that if your body senses you're starving, it does *everything it can to preserve your fat stores*.

I get cranky when I find they have cut all the fat off the meat (especially the bacon though its not good for you) as I love the taste, and it is naturally good for you to cook in its own fat rather than an oil.

We eat less fat than our ancestors, and our heart disease rates keep going up.

Saturated fats are a natural part of your diet, and they don't raise your risk of heart disease.

There are "good" saturated fats such as Lard, Butter, Beef tallow, Vegetables, eggs, coconuts and nuts.

FEET and TOES

Well, most of us at different times have foot problems in one way or another.

My small thin, flat feet have always been hard to fit shoes to, especially fashionable ones, and now I've graduated to needing some sort of orthotic. Also, they only bring in a few in my size, which means I either must warn the shop what I am looking for so they can ring when in, or in big shops I recently visited to get some cheap slippers they didn't even have any size 6 in most styles, or the few they brought in have gone.

Even if the size is right, I slide through them and not a lot of court shoes have existed in recent times.

I love shoes and want many colours and styles. I still have some 10 or more years old that are leather (now hardly available or extremely expensive), and they simply keep on keeping on. Not being in leather now cuts our contact to the earth's healing energy. Plastic and concrete cut us off.

When we are buying new shoes, in some way we are saying, "I'm moving in a new direction or want to". New beginnings. We want to put our "best foot forward". If we buy second-hand, we are to some extent, walking in another's shoes, i.e. life.

In India, sandals show the foot and if the second toe is bigger than the first the men say the women are likely to be too bossy. I've never thought I was but then I only have it on one foot.

Toes hold the ends of some meridians, so if you have a problem with your neck or head you could find your toes very sore. Massaging your foot can help the problem.

FINGERS and NAILS

Fingers can change shape over the years and people who read hands will tell you why. Certainly, we all have different finger prints and shaped fingers. I found having hand and palm readings have been spot on as to how I lead my life and feel, also our talents.

If your hand is clawing, this can be a lack of minerals, not arthritis which the doctor usually diagnoses. Certainly, I started to lose the use of one hand to pain and no strength, and I would drop things. I got onto the liquid colloidal minerals and it stopped.

Our bodies' meridians run from the head, down our arms and to our finger tips so using acupuncture and massaging in these areas can heal. This is why we can diagnose illness in our nails.

Nails

Our nails are very interesting and taken for granted until we have a problem.

They can warn us about out health though we don't know much about it. Best to go without nail polish to a doctor or naturopath for them to see the difference between the nails

When you look at your nails you will see there are curves, dips, ridges, and grooves. Check out how thick or thin they are and if your nails are chipped or broken. Make a note of the colour of the nail itself, the skin under it, and the skin around the nail.

You might notice changes over time. I think in recent years people are noticing their nails more as they are aware that under the nails can hold infections.

Healthy nails are pink with pinkish white moons. Most of my nails don't have moons.

Nails can be streaked, striped, bluish, whitish, dull, bending and chipped. It is wise to go to someone who understands the health issues you may have.

Thick nails that look a bit like claws are not natural and may mean an infection, fungal infection, allergic to medication and much more.

Split nails, which I'm inclined to have, are more about needing more vitamin C and protein.

Concave (spoon) nails can signal several internal issues, iron deficiency or too much iron, heart disease and more.

Pitted nails can be from banging up your hands, alopecia, psoriasis, zinc deficiency and more.

Ridges instead of smooth indicates something is wrong with your body. Don't just buff them up as they could be a warning of iron deficiency, lupus and inflammatory arthritis.

Dry, brittle nails – you don't need lotion or cuticle oil. If your nails are dry and brittle, you should check your hormone levels and bacterial health, thyroid.

Clubbed nails If you have plump skin that seems to swell around the nail, or if your nails seem to have puffed around your fingers, they are said to be "clubbed". Clubbed nails can mean liver, bowel or lung disease.

FISH

– see Cod-liver oil

Fish with the strongest omega 3 are salmon and mullet. Sardines are excellent and being tinned is fine if you don't want to work out how to cook them fresh. Heard on the radio about people who do Meals on Wheels, etc. finding a man who hadn't really had any meals for some time though he had been eating tinned sardines, and they found he was very healthy.

I find baking a whole fish, which can be stuffed with all sorts of herbs and spices, onions, garlic and tomato, is a delicious way to enjoy it. Fish be eaten fresh and at least once a week if not more.

It is preferable to buy fresh fish rather than farmed (in Australia most of our salmon and barramundi are farmed) and fed a range of foods that are not necessarily right for fish rather than natural sea food.

Unfortunately, in Tasmania, where they farm the salmon, the food has fallen to the bottom and caused a lot of pollution so maybe not such a good fish to have.

Truth about fish oil

Many tests from around the world have shown that:

Fish oil helps prevents second heart attacks better than any drug it was tested against!

Fish oil is probably the best "medicine" available to prevent sudden cardiac death!

Fish oil can be used if people can't take aspirin. If you don't like the taste, have some lemon or orange oil after to clear the taste. When I was young, I used to hold my nose.

It has been known to improve memory, IQ. and helps obliterate age-related memory lapses along with helping prevent strokes and high blood pressure.

Fish oil can be useful in treating prostate, breast and colon cancers. Because fish oil simultaneously improves hormone levels and improves the health of your joints, this makes it the perfect anti-ageing supplement as well as a superb supplement for athletes, speeding recovery time from hard workouts! Fish oil balances hormonal levels in the body, which has many benefits – one of which is a much sounder, deeper sleep, so that you wake up in the morning feeling totally refreshed and invigorated!

It is worth trying it for any health problems as it cuts inflammation and has no noticeable side effects.

FLU

– see Onions – Bicarb

Not a lot can be written on this subject unless I get into vaccination, which must be out of date as the flu differs every year. I have to say that most of my family and friends do not get vaccinated and don't get the flu, though they know of friends who get the vaccine every year and get the flu. The doctor tells them that the flu would have been much worse if they hadn't taken the vaccine. I wonder?

Much the same could be said of Covid 19.

If people eat good food and keep their immune system in order, they are unlikely to get the flu or any other infectious disease. Though I do know that if there is a lot of long-term emotional stress and trauma in a person's life, they are more vulnerable to the flu and most other illnesses.

Good food of course can mean lots of things to different people. Many don't realise they are eating food which is not good for them though they think it is. Often, for a start they are eating too much sugar, carbohydrates and too much food.

Many people are allergic to soy, dairy and wheat but think it is good for them. You do need to really check it out. Mostly they don't eat enough fruit and vegetables.

I think many call a bad cold "flu". One of my naturopaths considered it good to get a cold once a year to clean the body out.

FLUORIDE

For those not wanting to drink water because of the fluoride, you will find many articles on the internet. I use a water filter which takes the fluoride and chlorine out.

The problem called fluoridation

Around the world people most commonly encounter fluoride through water fluoridation and fluoridated toothpaste. Other sources include certain types of tea, pesticide residues in food, tobacco use, food cooked in non-stick teflon-coated cookware, medications and medical inhalers containing fluoridated gases.

Fluoride has no known essential function in human development, with no evidence of fluoride deficiency identified so far.

It has been commonly used to fight **dental caries.** I thought it strange back in the '60s to give the children I was looking after in UK a fluoride tablet before bed.

Fluoride is a by-product of the fertiliser industry that was added to municipal water treatment.

Claims of fluoride's role in preventing tooth decay can't be true as people who don't use it were having the same number of cavities.

Fluoride has been defected in tooth enamel caused by excess intake during the first 8 years of life and can permanently damage the enamel and clearly demonstrates toxicity in the body.

It has also been said to have a bad effect on the thyroid, teeth problems and many others.

In Australia, the US and a few other countries rate water fluoridation as one of the "top 10 public health achievements of the 20th century", but most of the Western world, including the vast majority of Western Europe, does not fluoridate its water supply.

Some countries fluoridate their salt the majority do not.

From my reading and television viewing, I have noticed a lot of tooth decay is now being found to come from too many sugar drinks, sugar generally and poor dental hygiene

Children's second teeth are often rotten. Doctors are now saying cut out the fruit juices, cordial, etc. and use water (cutting the sugar back helps the memory in children).

FORMALDEHYDE

This is found in carpets and many other products in new homes and factories.

I have included this chemical because I had many of these problems (continuing) while working in a carpet showroom with no fresh air coming in. I was unaware of this chemical and what it could do. In time I had this burning in the nose and face, red and inflamed, as I went upstairs to work. I was the only person there all day and sat under the air conditioner which no doubt circulated the fibres from the cut samples.

At last, I went to an ear, nose and throat doctor who said my septum was crooked (not a problem) and my nose was inflamed and it would probably be okay once I left the job. No talk about possible chemicals, etc.

I just had to leave, though little money and no job to go to and unaware of what was causing it. Today I would have sued (not my normal way of solving something) the company for the working conditions, mainly to pay for all the medical and natural things I've tried.

The right nostril where it meets my face is the problem area and it is where, many years ago, I had to have teeth out to get to cysts. I don't believe I have sinus problems as it shows clear when tested. More like there is something inside the flesh. I still suffer problems with my nasal area blocking at night and breathing. I was diagnosed at one time with Staph.

No dentist or doctor can see anything wrong. Massage and acupuncture help, but I can't do that all the time.

New houses can be very toxic and cause formaldehyde-exposure problems with people who are sensitive to the chemical. Exposure to it can cause all sorts of skin problems.

Long-term exposure to formaldehyde is reported to affect the central nervous system, causing headache, depression, mood changes, insomnia, irritability, attention deficit, impairment of dexterity, memory, and equilibrium.

Chronic exposure may be more serious for children because of their potential longer latency period.

I'm not blaming all my troubles on this, but I'm sure it was some of the problem.

FRUIT

– see Cancer – Heart – PH

Personally, I don't like mixing vegetable and fruit together. They sometimes seem to be contradictory. I like tropical fruits with each other: melons with melons and berries with their seasonal fruit etc. Originally my naturopath way back said melons should only be eaten together due to the effect it has with cleansing.

I will not do a whole list of fruit as it is easy for you to check on the internet, but this is general information and articles I have read on certain fruits.

It is well known that fruit is an important food and good for our whole system. Good fructose and fibre. Some can be used intensely to help our body when we have become ill from imbalances in our life.

Many people have reported healing cancer through changing their diets, way of life, clearing acidic foods, including eating fruit which can have a high pH up to 12. Especially using pineapple and pawpaw.

To reap the most benefits of pineapple (bromelain), consume it in juice form and incorporate other fruits so that you can take in more nutrients and vitamins and improve the taste.

For a start, try adding citrus fruits such as oranges, lemons, and limes to your pineapple juice. These fruits are known to boost immune function, and they're also anti-angiogenic, meaning that they reduce the growth of blood vessels which act as nutrient delivery mechanisms for cancer and tumours.

A suggested diet is:

- Days 1–7: all fruit diet with a beetroot-carrot-celery juice
- Days 8–10: same diet but no juice. Took vitamin K and sodium selenite (a form of selenium)
- Days 11–14: vegetables, soaked almonds, avocados, etc.

FRUITS SHOULD BE EATEN ON AN EMPTY STOMACH before meals. If you eat fruit like that, it will play a major role to detoxify your system, supplying you with a great deal of energy for weight loss and other life activities. With other food, you could be creating fermentation.

I have a meal of fruit most days (breakfast or lunch). I add protein by having a few spoons of a mix I do in bulk and keep in the freeze (various nuts and seeds ground up). Sometimes I add some goat/sheep yoghurt as well.

You have heard people complaining – "Every time I eat watermelon, I burp and when I eat durian, my stomach bloats, when I eat a banana, I want to run to the toilet, etc". All this will not arise if you eat the fruit on an empty stomach. The fruit mixes with the putrefying other food and produces gas, so you will bloat!

Greying hair, balding, nervous outburst and dark circles under the eyes – all these will NOT happen if you take fruits on an empty stomach.

Drink only fresh fruit juice, NOT from the cans, and don't drink juice that has been heated up. Drink it slowly to allow it to mix with your saliva.

Cooked fruits create some lack of the nutrients though of course it tastes good.

Eating a whole fruit is better than drinking the juice.

Just eat fruits and drink fruit juice throughout the 3 days and you will be surprised when your friends tell you how radiant you look. Though start with a couple of days of fasting and water.

Apple

An apple a day keeps the doctor away?

Although an apple has a low vitamin C content, it has antioxidants and flavonoids that enhance the activity of vitamin C, thereby helping to lower the risks of colon cancer, heart attack and stroke.

My mother grated it to have when we were ill and couldn't or didn't want to eat. Also, with a little orange juice it tasted great.

Apricot

About 40 years ago, I was told to take a teaspoon of apricot kernel oil once a day as a good preventative for cancer and keeps your copper level up, which is also good for slowing hair greying. I've done this on an off over the years.

It is known that the lifestyle habits of the Hunzas living in remote Northern Pakistan have great health, and many of them have lived for over 100 years.

Their vitality had a lot to do with what they eat and their overall lifestyle. Their diet is simple. Raw milk and occasional meat, bone broth, fresh grains and veggies. They eat very little sugar and their lifestyles as nomads and herders mean they get plenty of vigorous exercise.

The other characteristic is that the group eats large quantities of apricot seed kernels, which prove to be very healthy. If it comes to healing cancer, you would need to check the internet for the amount you would eat, etc.

Banana

Banana peel

It turns out that the biggest risk from a banana peel might really be slipping on it. The fact is, it's edible and packed with nutrients. It is eaten in many parts of the world, though it's not very common in the West.

High amounts of vitamin B6 and B12, as well as magnesium and potassium, are in the skin. It is important to carefully wash a banana peel before eating it due to the pesticides that may be sprayed in banana groves.

Never let it rot. When going off, peel it, break it off in bits and freeze in a large container. Use for smoothies or banana bread.

The peels are usually served cooked, boiled or fried, though they can be eaten raw or put in a blender with other fruits.

They are not as sweet as banana flesh. Riper peels will be sweeter than unripe ones.

Mashed banana is good for you when you don't feel well or don't want to eat.

To soothe an itchy bite, rub the inside of the peel across it.

Lightly rub scuffs on leather shoes with the inside of the peel, then wipe with a clean cloth. Scuffs gone.

Using the inside to rub over a dirty shower screen and wipe off creates a beautiful clean screen.

A friend uses the soft side as a patch on sores or bruises, she tapes it on with a Band-Aid.

Their soluble and insoluble fibre slows digestion, boosts feelings of fullness and helps lower cholesterol, all of which lead to weight loss.

Can be helpful for troubled sleep insomnia.

Banana use

It has been said do not put your banana in the refrigerator. I think this means the whole banana, not the skinned one.

Bananas contain 3 natural sugars – sucrose, fructose and glucose combined with fibre and it gives an instant, sustained and substantial boost of energy.

Research has proven that just 2 bananas provide enough energy for a strenuous 90-minute workout. No wonder the banana is the number one fruit of the world's leading athletes. A man in his 80s I know eats about 4 a day and though he has various diseases looks 10 years younger with plenty of energy for very long walks.

These are situations which have shown improvement:

Depression, premenstrual syndrome (PMS), anaemia, high blood pressure, constipation, hangovers, heartburn, morning sickness and mosquito bites affect the inside skin. Nerves, overweight, at-work ulcers, temperature control, seasonal affective disorder (SAD), smoking and tobacco use, stress, strokes and warts affect the skin.

Compared with apples, bananas have 4 times the protein, twice the carbohydrates, 3 times the phosphorous, 5 times the vitamin A and iron, and twice the other vitamins and minerals. It is also rich in potassium and one of the best value foods around.

Berries

I am not going to go into all the berries, only the ones I know a bit about.

Blueberries

Blueberries are just as healthy if frozen (up to 6 months) and could be described as one of the world's healthiest foods.

They go head to head with strawberries and pomegranates as antioxidants, great for eye protection and memory,

They have been used for heart, dementia, digestion – combating cancer, blood sugar and the nervous system.

Blueberries are one of our body's greatest allies. Their ability to eliminate free radicals protects us from everyday exposure to various forms of pollution, including pesticides, sun exposure and heavy metals.

Elderberry

For centuries they have been used to fight common infections, but interest has grown around them being used for its cold- and flu-reducing properties.

They are high in vitamins A, C, and E content, high levels of potassium, and its anti-inflammatory and antiseptic properties.

They are generally not available over the counter in Australia.

Strawberry

Strawberries are seasonal! And long loved for the fun of picking and the taste, but have drawn little attention for their health benefits. They are not, technically speaking, a berry. They belong to the pineapple family, having their seed on the outside.

They can be good for heart and possibly over-weight or obese people, provided they take a proper amount every day.

Also, as an antioxidant it is shown to help with osteoarthritis, cognition and blood-sugar control.

Grape

Eating grapes and other fruits rich in potassium has been shown to reduce rheumatoid arthritis symptoms, preventing painful gout attacks. They alkalise the blood and urine.

When the blood and urine are kept slightly alkaline, acid wastes are more easily eliminated, resulting in reduced at-tacks of rheumatoid arthritis symptoms and painful gout recurrences.

Recently I heard that people grill grapes, bake them and add them to other fruit and vegetables. They are good for a smoothie. Something I've never heard of.

The grape diet was developed in South Africa back in the '60s when people ate large meals of meat, then grapes and fruit afterwards. The rate of stomach cancer was consider-able and the person who developed the diet realised what was happening was due to fermentation.

You cleanse with only water for a few days, then you can eat grapes for every meal for a week and have some grape juice, if you wish, along with water of course. As grapes have many vitamins and minerals, you never feel weak or lacking in energy. You also don't feel hungry. Grapes can become boring, though.

The next week you incorporate other fruits and the week after add vegetables, then the week after meat if you wish. From then on only have fruit as a meal.

Certainly not after a meal.

Grapes also help prevent deposits in the joints of gout patients.

I followed this diet the first time when I wanted to lose weight after coming back from overseas in my 20s. Most of we Aussies put on weight in the UK due to television, which we hardly watched at home, the weather, biscuits, sweets and little exercise. I was not exactly a Twiggy, who my husband admired. Certainly lost a lot of weight. Don't know how much as didn't have scales in those days.

A friend of mine does the diet every year as a cleanse.

Grapefruit

It was first described as "forbidden fruit of Barbados" in the 18th century. However, grapefruit is packed full of nutrients and anti-cancer potential.

Grapefruit (Citrus paradisi or fruit of paradise) belongs to the citrus family of plants and is my favourite one of all citruses.

Guava

A lot of people don't know what Guava is or looks like. I had it first on Norfolk Island in the '60s, and they said it came with their deliveries from Northern New South Wales. This fruit is a clear winner for the high vitamin C content and is rich in fibre, which helps prevent constipation.

Kiwi fruit

They are tiny but mighty. A good source of potassium, magnesium, vitamin E and fibre. Its vitamin C content is twice that of an orange. It also is the only food that has zeaxanthin, which is needed for eye health.

Lemon-lime (Asian origin)

Some say lemon is 10,000 times stronger than chemotherapy. Use all the lemon you can.

Living in India in the '60s, we used to have lime-and-salt drink, which I loved, to make sure we didn't dehydrate. They also used juice and salt to clean copper. I had the drink again in Bali some years ago. I'm not sure of the actual recipe.

You can freeze a washed lemon and use it to grate on food, add to cooking and of course squeeze it for juice.

It is wonderful rubbing a squeezed half on your face. It may sting but that is only cleaning. After rinsing off, your face feels so smooth and soft.

For greasy, dirty hands, squeeze some juice in your cupped hand and add sugar (causes a sandpaper effect). Rub it all over and rinse off. You can also rub it on any sores as it will kill bugs.

Sore throat? Fill a small container or bottle with half lemon juice and half olive oil. Shaken, it creates a great mix to sip, which helps stop the coughing and sore throat. I used to take it to school with me.

Add the juice to the fresh water you drink. Make up a jug to remind you through the day to take water, gives nice taste and extra value.

Citrus delight is a wonderful dessert. Lemon is a summer-season favourite that typifies what it means to be a child. There used to be neighbourhood lemonade stands and warm, balmy days at the pool. But more than just a refreshing treat, lemon also contains a rich oil that science suggests could protect against certain types of cancer.

Native to the Middle East, lemon (or at least it's a modern variation), has gained considerable attention in scientific literature. It's been used to make everything from simple lemonade beverages and lemon liqueurs to vinegar and fermented healing elixirs. But perhaps its greatest potential is in essential oil form, which is where lemon really shines.

It has been used to stop human cervical cancer cells in their tracks.

A mixture of lemon essential oil and eucalyptus, melaleuca, lemongrass, clove leaf and thyme in a 40% ethanol base demonstrated anti-tumorigenic effects when administered to patients with metastatic tumorigenic ulcers. Cancer patients have also found relief from pain, anxiety, nausea, and vomiting by using lemon and other essential oils.

Orange

Orange is the sweetest medicine. Taking 2–4 oranges a day may help keep colds away, lower cholesterol, prevent and dissolve kidney stones as well as lessen the risk of colon cancer. However, this has been also known to have a bad liver effect on some people.

My son used to throw up at or just after parties as a child. My naturopath advised me to take him off chocolate and orange, especially not eaten at the same time. No problems.

Also, as a child we used to have the juice with a whipped-up raw egg yolk at breakfast sometimes. Another of the naturopath's suggestions. Delicious.

Papaya – see Pawpaw, Cancer

Papaya has been known to halt breast cancer and prostate cancer as it is full of cancer-fighting carotenoid and has a pH of 12 (alkaline). Enzymes from papaya digest proteins, including those that protect tumours.

In fact, it has been shown that eating most of the tree in one form or another helped cure cancer. Luckily, the people who did this lived in Queensland with lots of papaya/pawpaw available.

Have a slice of papaya every day. Papaya juice and ointment is also great and, to my shock the other day when cutting it up, I got it on my hand and fingers, which made them sting and itch. Must have been cleaning and clearing toxins so stayed with the pain for a while before I rinsed it off. Probably stimulated my circulation too. (Same happened with pineapple.) Never experienced it before.

Passionfruit

Being a dark red skin it is, like all red fruits and vegetables, good for the blood and heart (passion). I was told to use the skins simmered in water to help produce more blood as I tend to be low in blood content.

It got its name from the lovely shape of the flowers.

Great taste, of course, which many in Europe and Asia and Africa were not aware of, even in modern times. It is a native of Brazil, and most Australians would say Australia too as we all used to have them growing in the back yard. However, few are grown now at home and are therefore very expensive.

I remember at a painting group 15 years ago people brought in loads of them and we all got interested in the many recipes we could use to eat them. Great in icing.

Pawpaw
– see Papaya, Cancer

Megan Norris, wrote an article about how he father in Queensland with terminal lung cancer took pawpaw juice due to advice from locals who had been cured. So thought he'd give it a go. He planted 54 trees and would harvest leaves, with stems and boiled them, strained them and put the juice in a glass jar in the fridge. He drank 250 ml 3 times a day.

Her mother decided to help with iron so got 500 g fresh calves liver and squeezed it to make a pulp then mixed it with vegie juice in the processor and gave 250 mil to him with a quarter of orange. Luckily he was prepared to take it though it had a dreadful taste.

The Cancer improved in quite a short time to every-one's amazement.

Pineapple
– see Cancer

My main experience apart from pineapple being delicious in fruit salad, etc. is related to a throat infection.

My herbalist had suggested this and it has proved to be a winner in clearing up a yellow infected throat. Years later when I used the freshly ground juice of a pineapple for my brother to gargle with it and spit it out, the results were amazing. We spaced it out over an hour or so to use up all the pineapple. I was amazed at the completely clear throat.

Another time, my son had been very sick, sore throat and unable to get up in the morning. He rang for help so I took my pineapple and juicer over went through the ritual and went home. In the evening I rang him to see how he was, and he was so good he was out partying!

Pineapple is high in vitamins, minerals, phosphorus and magnesium, which are all needed for good health and immunity as its pH is about 12 (alkaline)

Lots of enzymes are in bromelain (whole pineapple), which are anti-inflammatory.

It can relieve joint pain from gout and most types of arthritis and fibromyalgia, relieves sore throats, stops the development of new tumors and shrinks existing cancers, reduces post-operative swelling, eliminates acid reflux, and supplies enzymes to promote and speed digestion and motility of the bowel and much more.

So, "If you like Pina Coladas and getting caught in the rain, or not, and, whether you're into yoga or Sunday afternoon football, if you have half a brain", you'll add pineapple to your diet to take advantage of their myriad of health benefits and tastiness.

Pomegranate

Pomegranate is found to help prevent coronary artery disease progression, also ideal for many women's diseases.

Modern women at midlife have many options when it comes to dealing with those nasty menopausal symptoms like mood swings, depression, bone loss, and fluctuating oestrogen levels, and this has proved to be helpful

It can be helpful for bone loss, mood improvement and heart health.

Pomegranates have been cultivated for over 4,000 years. Our word "pomegranate" dates to around 750 BC and comes from the Latin "Panicum malum", meaning "Phoenician apple." Today the fruit is often called a "Chinese apple."

Bit hard to work out how to eat them. I cut in half and bend them back so the seeds pop out but still messy though delicious. Juice is now available in shops.

Tamarind
– see Cholesterol

People continue to sound the alarm about fluoride, which is linked with debilitating bone disease, low thyroid function, reduced IQ, infertility and various forms of cancer. For natural health, a unique fruit is gaining the attention of researchers for its fluoride-detoxifying properties.

It is helpful with cholesterol and diabetes.

Tamarind is used all over the Middle East, India and Asia, but in Australia the fruits (without the seeds) are available from Chinese and Indian supermarkets. It is often in jars but the slabs can be found as well, which is what I use for health. Many people from overseas already know the tamarind as it is used in drinks and food recipes.

With the drug scares happening regularly and statin drugs being reported to cause severe problems and death, it is worthwhile to recognise the benefits of tamarind, nutmeg and mustard, all of which will reduce cholesterol levels quickly.

However, cholesterol is made in the body to protect our arteries at a time when they show decline.

Tamarind is very strong in vitamin C and lysine, according to Linus Pauling, the famous Nobel Prize winner (twice), 3 grams each a day of vitamin C will prevent damage to arteries and the body's need to make life-saving cholesterol.

Tamarind recipe used for cholesterol:

Remove all the fruit from the packet (slab), add water and boil. (Slabs used to be 8 oz then 4 oz.) My notes show 4 litres of water for 8 oz, which from memory lasted for 2 weeks. Haven't done it for a few years so not sure. Hold a strainer over a big container to get the juice, and you can use the fruit for cooking.

Let it stand until cool enough to drink and take 1 glass a day. Keep the rest in a glass bottle in the fridge and drink hot or cold.

Never use a microwave to heat or cook!!

My cholesterol went right down within a few months, maybe sooner, but I didn't check earlier.

Watermelon

It is the coolest thirst quencher. Composed of 92% water, nutrients found in watermelon are vitamin C and potassium. It is best eaten with other melons as they work together. Some fruits lose their value or cause problems when mixed with incompatible ones.

As it is mostly water, try and find organic watermelon if possible as it absorbs so much moisture from the soil.

My children got a sort of foot-and-mouth illness and the only thing they would/could eat was watermelon. Everything else stung.

FUNGI

– see Mould, Mushrooms

Fungi is known as one of the biggest killers in the world in one form or another.

Animals, bats, etc. can spread it and once in the food, like the potato famine in Ireland in the 1840s showed just how devastating such pathogens can be.

Look to some of the natural cures for fungi on the body like tea tree, oil of cloves, oxygen and hydrogen peroxide.

Many people die from it being inside their body. It seems to be hard to diagnose once in there and if found in time the person can be healed. I'm inclined to think that by having a teaspoon of bicarb soda in water every day it would not thrive.

G

GARDASIL

– see Vaccine, HPV

Gardasil was developed for the STD known as HPV and was approved by the FDA (Food and Drug Administration) in 2006. The disease was not of concern until the 1980s. It was mainly aimed at preventing the HPV which form in the cervix, and it can cause cancer if women don't have their regular check-up.

The Gardasil vaccine is being given to teenage girls and now going to boys. The push is on to get the boys as well to prevent anal and penile cancer. Very few people get these cancers, so it doesn't seem necessary given the terrible consequences of having the vaccine.

Many girls have died or been damaged in the heart for life, and in various forms, not long after the shot, in some places, parents aren't asked if they allow it. It is given through the schools.

Here are the ingredients of the HPV vaccine, Gardasil:

- sodium borate (borax)
- 225 ug amorphous aluminium hydroxy phosphate sulphate
- polysorbate 80
- L-histidine hydrochloride
- 4 recombinant VLP's: HPV types – 16, 18, 11 and 6
- amino Acids, carbohydrates, mineral salts, vitamins

Sodium borate and polysorbate 80 are known to cause infertility in laboratory rats.

There are now reports coming in that girls who took Gardasil are finding it hard to get pregnant, and Silica cell salts are having some effect in drawing out the metals used in the vaccine.

GM – GENETICALLY MODIFIED FOOD

Food grown with genetically modifying chemicals cannot reproduce, so farmers can't keep some seeds from one year to plant in the next. They must buy new seeds. This means thousands of farmers in India and other places have committed agricultural suicide because it is too expensive to keep buying seeds. So they have nothing to grow the next year and therefore no food.

This is probably true of many places. Many garden seeds today are hybrid and therefore unable to reproduce. If food isn't alive to regrow, it can't be good for our bodies. Also, with GM someone is holding power over our choice of nourishment.

If it gets into organic fields next door, the people can't sell their organic food as it can't be cleared of the GM.

Several seed stores have been set up by people to hold seeds for all foods and people can buy the real seed. I've been suggesting people buy some now in case there is a rush on them. There is a huge amazing Seed store built in an icy place by Bill Gates.

GOUT

– see Bicarb, Baking soda, Grapes

GRANDMA'S CURES

(no guarantee they work) and HEALTH HINTS

Cure urinary tract infections with Alka-Seltzer … Just dissolve 2 tablets in a glass of water and drink it at the onset of the symptoms. Alka-Seltzer begins eliminating urinary tract infections almost instantly – even though the product has never been advertised for this use.

Honey remedy for skin blemishes … Cover the blemish with a dab of honey and place a Band-Aid over it. Honey kills the bacteria, keeps the skin sterile and speeds healing. Works overnight.

Listerine therapy for toenail fungus … Get rid of unsightly toenail fungus by soaking your toes in Listerine mouthwash.

The powerful antiseptic leaves your toenails looking healthy again.

Tea tree oil … Put quite a lot in a spray with water as your pest spray. They can't breathe and drop dead. Good to spray all around where the cupboards meet the floor. Smells nice and fresh and doesn't stain if sprayed on fabric. Also put on fungal nails and the start of a cold sore.

Easy eyeglass protection … To prevent the screws in eyeglasses from loosening, apply a small drop of clear nail polish to the threads of the screws before tightening them.

Cleaning liquid that doubles as a bug killer … If menacing bees, wasps, hornets get into your home and you can't find the insecticide, try a spray of cleaning fluid. Insects drop to the ground instantly.

Smart splinter remover … Just pour a drop of glue over the splinter, let dry and peel the dried glue off the skin. The splinter sticks to the dried glue.

Sun lotion contains aluminium nanoparticles, which are more dangerous to the brain than larger particles. It also ends up in the sea when swimming, which adds to all the other particles entering the sea. Fish eat contaminated food, birds eat it, and we end up eating it. Universities are doing research in Sydney Harbour, and it seems we are poisoning the whole world with nanoparticles. It is also a problem for coral.

Acne

Coconut oil rubbed in can be very helpful.

Sugar

Dulls the brain, making it hard to learn and remember, stimulates appetite (hungry all the time), colds and causes restlessness.

Itches can be stopped by spraying on colloidal silver.

Itching and stinging in your legs after a bath is caused by circulation. Either get into bed and cover up or use something like a dry towel, throw or whatever to cover the area. The warmth does the trick. I had it often as a child (due to my heart problem) so avoided the bath.

Iodine

Keep in the house for cuts, etc.

Bicarb soda

Can beat cancer.

Birth pain

Pain threshold equals 20 bones getting fractured at the same time.

Cough/colds

Peel and chop one red onion place in a bowel and drizzle honey over it. Cover with wrap or a tea towel, leave overnight. Then strain the onion from the syrup. Take one tablespoon of cough mixture every 2 hours (children, one teaspoon every 2 hours).

Squeeze a lemon and put an equal amount of olive oil in. Sip this through the day, especially before going to bed. It really soothes the throat.

Make a warm drink out of lemon juice, honey, chilli, garlic and ginger. Excellent for healing colds.

PH Factor – low pH = very acidic – high = alkaline. Ranges between 4 – 8 Can be seen in a ribbon you can get at health-food shops. Spit into an egg cup and then run a bit of the ribbon through it. Five and below shows poor immunity to many diseases. Pineapple and pawpaw are off the list at 12–14 so great for healing.

Coffee and cancer have the same pH factor or 4.5.

Diarrhoea

Ginger oil – 4–5 drops in water relieves.

Ear aches/infections

Peroxide 3% is okay to use undiluted for earaches and infection/cuts. A teaspoon of it in the ear, allow to bubble up then turn to side and let it out.

Stings (wasp etc) or itches (eczema etc)

Spray-on colloidal silver. You can buy this in a health-food shop, in a glass bottle with spray top. Stops the itch or pain immediately. You can also make your own as it can be expensive.

Emotional health

To resolve stressful situations, especially in relation-ships we need to:

Heal the physical – material – emotional – mental – spiritual which means lots of research, reading and practising.

Relationship book guru – Harvel Hendriks has written at least 3 books. He and his wife run a worldwide organisation called Imago.

Five happy positive comments counteract one negative critical one. A person can handle the critical one and rela-tionship is happy.

Five critical, negative comments to one positive comment creates an unhappy relationship, eventually destroying it.

GREEN TEA

Green tea can be sipped with meals as it is good for diges-tion. Suggest you check the net for more details as it also good for healing and preventing other problems.

GRIEF

– see Death and Dying

There are several books on this subject, as discussed in the other subjects.

GUMS

– see Dental

If swollen gums are deep red, sensitive to brushing, and easily bleed, it is a mild form of gum disease known as gingivitis. If left untreated, gingivitis can manifest into peri-odontitis, which is inflammation around the teeth that cause the gums to pull away from the teeth. This creates pockets between the teeth and the gums that is the perfect envi-ronment for bacteria to proliferate. When the bacteria and plaque spread below the gum line, bone, connective tissue and gum tissue starts to break down.

Check with your herbalist or holistic dentist what to use to heal.

Coconut oil held in the mouth for 5 minutes or so will help reduce inflammation.

For any problems I have with my gums like ulcer or swelling, etc., I swear by myrrh. I know it is supposed to be mixed with water, but I put some on my finger and rub it in gently. Usually, it is healed within a day or so.

Myrrh is also great to put in your face cream, just a few drops mixed in. I have suggested it to people with haemorrhoids as it heals in the wet mouth so could well do the same round the anus.

GUT

There is a huge amount of information on the net regarding the gut and digestion, as well as how it can affect the whole body when infected or bloated. Sometimes the walls of the gut can become weakened and bacteria can seep through.

My naturopath at one time said the first thing to fix with a person who has a major disease like cancer is to get the gut working properly as it is the seat of all digestion.

When I had a bit of seepage, she said to get an organic chicken, simmer the chicken bones for a long time, then make a broth. I think I just had that for a few days on rice. It was a special type of rice which I think was organic. Could add a bit of tahini paste, rather than soy sauce. Maybe needs more research.

H

HAIR
– see FACE AND HAIR

HEADACHE
– MIGRAINE

Headaches can be caused by many health problems, and they often affect different parts of the head. Our meridians that go from head to toe affect all the organs.

First and foremost, if these suggestions don't work within a day or so, go to the doctor as it may be something much more complicated.

I read an article by a doctor some time ago who found her migraines came at a regular time in the month as mine often did (acupuncture worked for my migraine). She also had irregular periods so she left a light on in the bedroom in the middle of the month for a few nights, which seemed to do the trick in keeping her periods regular.

Headaches from stress can be helped by pressing your fingers into the area of muscle between your thumb and first finger. If it is painful, massage it until it is not hurting, and you can find your headache is relieved.

Migraines are usually found in people who contain/supress their anger and feelings, mostly women or men who are more the gentle type like Cancer, Pisces, Libra. Also stress, dehydration and poor posture can all help to create it.

I've found fiery type personalities, including women, rarely get them.

In astrology, Mars (male) rules the head and it is common for men to complain that their wife doesn't want sex because she has a headache. I found that happened to me once, not wanting sex because of a headache, but as I hadn't seen my boyfriend for some time, we went ahead. The last thing I wanted. However, my headache disappeared. The stress and frustration was released. Bounced out of bed full of energy, whereas before I was wilting on the lounge.

Once visiting my sister and going down with a headache/ migraine, she started to massage my head and neck while I had a drink of water and then I slowly nibbled on some dry biscuits, though I didn't feel I could eat anything. Shows how the sugars in our system can work. Too low or too high. I was fine after a while.

Recently I have found when dizzy (which happens quite a bit) I get up from the computer, stretch my neck and shoulders and drink about 2 glasses of water, do some deep breathing and eat a snack. I feel OK. Nuts and dried fruit are a good snack.

If really bad though and I feel dizzy, no energy and nausea, I go to acupuncture to balance the ying and yang or stop the chi from stagnating.

HEART

– see Cayenne Pepper, Blood pressure, Breath, Strawberries, Water, Fruit

Heart transplant

It has been found that people who had a transplant developed a whole lot of likes and dislikes that were completely new to them. After checking with families as to what tastes, etc. the family were aware of, it seems some had developed these changes due to the person whose heart it was.

Heart attack

It is best to drink warm water about a half hour after a meal, also go for a walk or wait quite a while to allow the digestion of a baked dinner, etc. before bed. This can help avoid a heart attack. In fact, at one of my Reiki workshops, the nurses doing the course said that heart attacks often happened at night after a big meal. Heart attack is one of the main killers of women. You may never have a chest pain during a heart attack. Nausea and intense sweating are also common symptoms.

Sixty per cent of people who have a heart attack while they are asleep do not wake up. Luckily, a pain in the jaw can wake you from a sound sleep.

If you are having pains on a regular basis in your back near the heart or down your arms, though you seem to be clear of a heart problem, you are worried. I go for a massage and/or acupuncture to release the tension in the nerve area around the heart and down the arm which when left can eventually lead to a heart problem. This is something I do on a regular basis, as sometimes I think I'm having a heart attack and go to the doctor only to get the all clear. Time after time.

Take an aspirin at night so it remains strongest overnight, which is a common time to have a heart attack.

Have to say as a child (with a heart murmur) I used to climb up and get them out of the medicine cupboard because I like the taste. Maybe it was a help. I now keep mine in the drawer beside the bed. Not that I use them much but I still get worried about my heart (childhood fear of dying).

HEMP
– see Cannabis

I you haven't tried hemp seeds as a regular part of your diet, you might want to try them. They can be enjoyed in cereals, granola, salad dressings, desserts and make a wonderful dairy-free milk.

They contain a vast number of vitamins, zinc and much more.

Hemp oil is now considered to be very good for all kinds of skin and health problems. It is of course related to cannabis

HERBAL CREAMS
– see Bruises and sprains

Arnica

This cream stops bruising and inflammation, especially if applied immediately. One of my childhood cures. However, we used the tincture which you can't buy over the counter now.

Chickweed

People have told me that chickweed is growing everywhere. I don't know what it looks like but they have found it is good for skin-cancer spots.

It is also good for eczema and psoriasis.

Rosemary massage cream

Has been successful for joint pain for bad knees and wrists. Also, for arthritic pain and poor circulation.

Comfrey cream

Another one used in childhood. It can mend bones in half the time, among other things, originally called "knit bone". The government banned the liquid, which acted more quickly, as someone had bad effects from it.

Before that, I suggested using the medicine to a friend who had broken her shoulder. The doctor was mystified that it took about half the usual time.

It is good for ulcerated skin, dry skin and dermatitis.

Elder-leaf liniment

Massage it in to injuries and it can be almost pain free.

It can be good for sprains and bruises, eczema and dermatitis.

Herbal lip balm

Helps stops wrinkles round lips, good for herpes simplex.

I always find tea tree oil stops herpes too.

Herbal foot balm

Use it for athlete's foot and great for fungal toe nail.

I find tea tree oil does wonders too for fungal toe nail. Works quite quickly.

HERBS and SPICES

I will only be covering the ones I have information on but suggest you check the others on the internet.

Probably cayenne, garlic, oregano and turmeric (organic if possible) are the most well known to help fight cancer. They are used every day in large amounts in cooking, sprinkled on food.

Cayenne pepper contains capsaicin, which burns our mouth, etc. This is the stuff that kills cancer cells. It has been called a cure-all herb but most of all very good for the heart. It has been known to stop a heart attack instantly and if you have heart problems you might be better off taking cayenne daily instead of drugs.

Garlic

Garlic is a very powerful anti-cancer spice. Studies all over the world have shown it to lower the risk of developing all types of cancers, especially colon, stomach, intestinal, and prostate cancer.

The World Health Organization recommends adults have a daily dose of fresh garlic (approximately one clove).

Garlic-and-lemon cleanse

This cleanse dissolves the plaque in the arteries and veins of the heart and will clear all blockages, so perhaps good for your nose/face. It improves vision and mental alertness.

> 30 cloves of (organic) garlic, peeled
>
> 5 diced fresh (organic) lemons, not peeled
>
> 1 litre of filtered water.

Place garlic and lemon chopped in a food processor and mince up (don't make it too mushy!). Bring mixture to gentle boil in the litre of water and remove immediately from heat. Strain, let it cool and then bottle in glass, to be kept in the fridge.

A daily dose of one liqueur glass (30 ml) may be taken either before or after the main meal of the day.

After having enjoyed this daily intake for 6 weeks, you will already notice a youthfully comfortable energetic whole body with less mucus, assured by supporters of this regime. The plaque deposits, and their side effects on sight and hearing for example, will start to vanish altogether. After 6 weeks, have a break for 8 days and then commence the second 6-week treatment for more success.

This therapeutic course of treatment should be repeated once a year.

The left-over garlic and lemon can be used in all sorts of cooking so nothing is wasted. It doesn't go off so can be kept for a long time.

Garlic has been used the world over for wonderful taste and for healing colds. A friend of mine from Europe back in the '50s said they used to hang it round their necks on a string to prevent infections. It is also a natural detoxifier of lead and much more.

For many years I have used garlic capsules taking 4 capsules x 4 times a day when I have a cold. Also, fresh garlic and onion sandwiches are delicious. The first time I did it, I had had bronchitis for 6 months, and it cleared up very quickly.

When in Bali I went down with a cold and coughing from the flight. In the local café, they have a drink especially for that. It has fresh garlic, ginger, chilli chopped up in a big drink of warm lemon juice with honey. My family uses it now and find it clears colds quickly.

Oregano has extremely high levels of antioxidants and antimicrobial compounds. It also contains vitamin K and iron. Lately there are oregano pills and oil. Good to take when travelling.

Turmeric is an anti-inflammatory, and it contains the powerful cancer-fighting polyphenol, curcumin, which has been clinically shown to inhibit growth of various cancer cells.

Drug-resistant infections are expected to kill more people than cancer by 2050. Thousands every year are already getting antibiotic-resistant infections and die. Staph is a problem in hospitals where people didn't have it when they went in.

The more they're prescribed weakened biotics, the worse the problem is getting.

Ayurvedic doctors consider curcumin to be a cure-all. Its antibiotic action kills bacteria to prevent infection and relieves pain and inflammation.

Suggest you make a paste to use for healing a stubborn wound:

- Mix 1 to 2 teaspoons ground turmeric with enough water or coconut oil to make a thick paste.
- Apply the paste to the wound and cover with a bandage. Let sit for at least 12 hours, and up to 24. Do this for 3 days.

Curry powder

A common ingredient in Indian and Asian cuisine, which is typically a mixture of coriander, turmeric, cumin, fenugreek and red pepper. This would be in a lot of Indian food so a good preventer of health problems.

Cinnamon

Of significant importance is cinnamon's ability to reduce tumour growth. Essential oil of cinnamon has been shown to suppress the growth-cell factors in carcinoma cells.

Cloves

Some people have managed to clear the mould in the house with oil of cloves. I put it in a spray with water, but didn't seem to work for me. Probably need to get the exact mix.

Back years ago, it was used for toothache by rubbing it in and around the tooth.

Like many of the herbs and spices it is also shown to be helpful in stopping cancer-cell growth by applying it to the cells on the skin

Curcumin
– see Turmeric

Curcumin, when given in combination with drugs for lung cancer, can reduce the cancer. Shortness of breath, a hoarse voice, and persistent cough are warning signs you shouldn't ignore. They're the most common signs of lung cancer.

Curcumin is also a boon for those suffering from various aches and pains. It helps lift the burden of arthritis sufferers and those with diverticular disease, irritable bowel (IBS), inflammatory bowel disease, dyspepsia and peptic ulcer because it protects the stomach lining.

Curcumin
– black seed oil

This oil is very good for all skin problems.

For asthma and bronchial problems

Mix a teaspoon of black seed oil in coffee. Take twice daily. Also rub your chest with black seed oil every night and inhale the vapour of black seed oil in hot water.

Backache and other kinds of rheumatism

Mildly heat a small amount of black seed oil and then stroke the rheumatic area intensely. A teaspoon of the oil should also be drunk 3 times daily.

Diabetes

Mix a cup of whole black seeds, a cup of watercress or mustard seeds, half a cup of pomegranate peel, and half a cup of fumitory (Ayurvedic medicine). Grind the mixture to powder. Take half a teaspoon of the mixture together with a teaspoon of black seed oil daily before breakfast for one month.

Diarrhea

Mix a teaspoon of black seed oil with a cup of yoghurt. Drink the mixture twice a day until symptoms disappear.

Dry cough

A teaspoon of black seed oil should be mixed in coffee and taken twice a day. Rub the chest and back with black seed oil. (My Chinese medicine man says it is from the liver and drink lots of water.)

Flu and nasal congestion

Placing 3 to 4 drops of black seed oil in each nostril can relieve nasal congestion and head cold distress.

Hair greying

Massaging the hair with black seed oil regularly may prevent premature hair greying.

Hair Loss

Stroke the scalp thoroughly with lemon and leave for about 15 minutes, shampoo, wash and dry hair thoroughly. Then massage black seed oil into the scalp. Drink a teaspoon of black seed oil mixed in tea/coffee.

Headaches

Rub the forehead and the sides of the face near the ears with black seed oil and bandage the head. Also, a teaspoon of black seed oil should be taken before breakfast.

Healthy being

To maintain good health, take a teaspoon of black seed oil mixed with one teaspoon of pure honey, twice daily.

Healthy complexion

Mix a tablespoon of black seed oil with a tablespoon of olive oil. Rub the face with this mixture and leave it for at least one hour. Wash with natural soap and water.

Flaxseed

This oil doesn't go rancid and therefore used for cooking. I use it to oil my chopping board.

Gingko Biloba

Ginkgo biloba, is one of the oldest-living tree species and best-selling herbs. It also protects the brain from the toxic effects of aluminium-chloride exposure, which has been linked to diseases such as Alzheimer's and other cognitive impairments.

Many have found it combined with bilberry excellent for aged macular degeneration and the mental functioning of Alzheimer's patients.

Hypertension

Mix any drink with a teaspoon of black seed oil and also take 2 lobes of garlic every morning with breakfast. Rub all the body with black seed oil and expose your body to sun rays for half an hour once every 3 days. Repeat for one month.

Laziness and fatigue

One tablespoon of black seed oil with a glass of pure orange juice every morning for at least 10 days.

Memory improvement

A teaspoon of black seed oil mixed in 100 mg of boiled mint for at least 15 days.

Muscular pains

Massage the area with black seed oil.

Ginger

Travel sickness – Ginger pills called Travacalm can be bought in a health-food shop/chemist shop, brilliant for sea sickness which I am prone to. I've proved it time after time. Though in the past I got sea sick very easily just sitting in a small rocking boat.

A friend and I went on a whale-watching trip and took a pill each once we got on the boat. People were throwing up all over the place, and we were fine.

At sea, I was fine for a couple of days but when I went below to iron I started to feel quite nauseous. Never mind the ironing. I took a pill and stayed up where the fresh air was. I remember when I was first on a ship going overseas in the '60s the only advice I got when it started rolling in the Atlantic was "Don't look at the horizon and sip a brandy". It was helpful. Didn't know about ginger pills then.

It is also ideal to take on the plane to avoid a sick bag and when travelling on winding roads, which can have a bad effect on you. Can't always know of course when a winding road might turn up.

Ginger and lemon are considered by several tests to be much, much stronger than chemo in targeting cancer.

This flowering plant also contains potent anti-inflammatory compounds called gingerols, a substance that can help reduce pain in people with osteoarthritis and rheumatoid arthritis, even improving their mobility when consumed regularly.

It's clear that ginger has amazing healing capabilities like those of turmeric. It's another one of those herbs that work both medicinally and as a staple in many fine-tasting cuisines.

Ginger is incredibly versatile, as it can be used in both sweet and savoury food.

Luckily, keeping fresh ginger around a house is a lot easier than you might think. This herb is super easy and low maintenance to grow with wonderful flowers.

Conditions that ginger absolutely loves are a sheltered spot to grow, filtered sunlight, warm weather, humidity, and rich, moist and loose soil. It does not thrive well in frosts, direct sunlight, strong winds or soggy, waterlogged soil.

Best way to start it is to get a piece from the supermarket and soak it in water overnight, as it may have been treated with a growth retardant. However, if you get some from a friend, let it dry for 24–48 hours before planting into a medium-sized, well-draining pot.

Best to plant ginger in the late winter or early spring where it's protected from wind and can receive indirect sunlight. Mature ginger requires 8 to 10 months of growing. However, some say you can begin stealing tiny bits of root around 4 months. The best time to harvest is when the leaves die down.

Lemon Grass

Lemon grass eaten or made into a drink has proved to be successful in attacking cancer cells.

An Israeli farmer was amazed that so many people with cancer were turning up asking for fresh lemon grass. Turned out their doctor had sent them.

They had been told to drink 8 glasses of hot water with fresh lemon grass steeped in it on the days that they went for their radiation and chemotherapy treatments.

It all began when researchers at Ben Gurion University of the Negev discovered that the lemon aroma in herbs like lemon grass kills cancer cells in vitro, while leaving healthy cells unharmed though they didn't know why.

Mint

There are several varieties of mint. Again, it is not just a lovely decorative aroma with a fresh taste.

Some varieties have properties that defend against cancer. It can be helpful for sufferers of irritable bowel syndrome.

Mint also provides many essential minerals such as calcium, copper, fluoride, iron, potassium, selenium, and zinc. The essential oils found in mint include menthol, menthone, and menthol acetate.

Parsley

Parsley is a natural vitamin and mineral which people found was decorative and tasty when in foods.

It is in fact, packed with so many nutrients that eating it is almost like taking a multivitamin and mineral supplement. Therefore, it has a positive effect on most health problems.

It is a high-chlorophyll blood purifier that aids in detoxification, particularly of the kidneys, but also of the liver. And the herb packs in dense nutrients, including vitamin A, vitamin C, beta-carotene, calcium, magnesium, phosphorus, iron, manganese, potassium, folic acid, sulphur, vitamin K, and B vitamins 1, 2, 3, 5, and 6.

I remember as a child; people would juice a big amount which you need (most people grew it in their garden along with mint) to give more iron when people were anaemic.

Parsley was one of the top 4 herbs revealed to have the highest inhibitory effects on cancer-inducing inflammatory compounds.

Peppermint

Peppermint is a member of the mint family. A favourite herbal medicine of the ancients, peppermint leaves have been found in Egyptian pyramids dating back to 1000 BC.

It is native to the Mediterranean and nutrient-rich. The fresh herb contains ample amounts of vitamins A, C, B12, K, along with folic acid, thiamine and riboflavin.

Most of us have experienced peppermint as a flavouring agent, or perhaps as a comforting cup of herbal tea, but are unaware of its wide range of experimentally confirmed therapeutic properties.

Radium weed
– Cansema

Many years ago, in the bush it was well known that radium weed was squeezed on a skin cancer, it would drop off.

Seems if cansema is advertised as a cure you can be fined or even sent to jail. Obviously, the big pharma companies don't want something simple like that to work as there is no money in it.

Rosemary

As mentioned before, so many herbs have both a cooking and medical use. Great with roast chicken or lamb.

Rosemary is good for eye health and may even protect against age-related macular degeneration, which is deterioration of the central area of the retina resulting in blind spots (my situation is discussed at the start of this book).

Rosemary is also used worldwide as a symbol of remembrance and it is good for memory so use the essential oil and herbal tea on a regular basis along with sage.

Sage

Sage has been known to sharpen memory in a few hours. It's interesting to note that a wise person is called a sage.

In 1597, herbalist John Gerard proclaimed that sage "is singularly good for the head and brain and quicken the nerves and memory." In 1652, Nicholas Culpeper advised, "It also heals the memory, warming and quickening the senses."

Some people have been tested with around 50 mg and 150 mg of sage oil which sharpens the memory in a few hours. So it looks as if it could help with dementia or Alzheimer's disease,

I was having some serious memory problems. Finding things in the most unlikely place and often having to ask others what something was called if I described it. So, after reading an article about sage mixture being great for memory, I have been using sage tea every day, and I am noticing quite an improvement. I do have it growing, so use it when I use a herb mixture for cooking.

I had an appointment with my acupuncturist, herbalist and neuro worker one day, and in the morning, I completely lost my memory when driving. Finding myself in some strange place. Then terrified that I might have to change my whole lifestyle and not drive in future.

I was amazed that in testing me, he said, "Your left brain is not talking to your right brain". He did some more work on me, and I've not had a memory problem in a year or more. Though I am finding again, a lot more, that I can't remember the name of some things. I know them if someone says the words or some time later. Seems it is only part of aging and normal.

Thyme

Studies have found that the super-herb, thyme essential oil, potently kills lung- and breast cancer cells.

Fresh thyme also makes a great addition to a healthy diet focused on organic fruits, vegetables and can be used as a tea.

HERTZ SOUND

– see Water – Ears

Sound has been known for years to affect our health and hearing.

Read the book by Patricia and Rafaele Joudry on **Sound Therapy Healing (1999).**

The book is based on the work of Dr Tomatis from France, who discovered the effect the various hertz had on the actual ear and how a therapy is used at a certain hertz to heal or improve tinnitus, hearing, autism and many other problems including eyesight.

HERTZ VIBRATION

369 Hz	turns grief to joy
417 hz	cleanses traumas, helps change
432 hz	great healer music by Mozart, Beethoven, etc.
440 Hz	**Hitler changed to this from 432** as have others to help numb the people.
520 Hz	natural earth, repairs DNA
639 Hz	communication
741 hz	power of self-expression
852 hz	awakens intuition
963 hz	restore spirit, light or God. To restore sleep, use in the background.

Boom-boom rock builds up tension with no roll to release it, whereas rock and roll goes up and down to a rhythm, which is not harmful. Classical music is the best music to study by.

As we are 70% water, we absorb everything by vibration. Dr Emoto found dirty cloudy water crystals came from 440 Hz and nasty-thoughts vibration. Whereas using 432 Hz and people sending love, beautiful crystals appeared.

HOMEOPATHY

I was amazed and delighted that when I was in France, I found almost every chemist shop had a section for homeopathy, and you could choose who you wanted to see – a homeopath or doctor. Homeopathy is also commonly used in various other countries, especially in Germany and Switzerland. Doctors prescribe homeopathy as well as Western medicine, depending on the problem.

Sadly, strong evidence of bias against homeopathy and many other natural therapies is shown by big pharma, and I have to say now it has become apparent that Wikipedia no longer shows the truth on many subjects. There is a lot of misinformation on natural health remedies, which scares people off

At least 100 million people in India use homeopathic and Ayurvedic medicines for ALL of their health care needs.

Living in Calcutta, I was fascinated to see a large hospital. At one end it was homeopathic, the middle was a mixture of Indian and Western, and the other end was all Western medicine. To me that is how it should be. I also found it hard to find a good natural therapist as everyone naturally told me to use the top local doctors. I wouldn't know how to find one then but being in my 20s didn't push it.

Though the positive efficacy of homeopathic medicines has been published in many of the most respected medical journals in the world, including *The Lancet*, *British Medical Journal*, *Chest* (the publication of the American College of Chest Physicians) and many others, it doesn't get to the public.

Ninety-two per cent of doctors working with top German football (soccer) teams prescribe homeopathic medicines for the players.

Significant support for homeopathy, acupuncture and other natural forms of healing has been shown to be of interest by medical students in Brazil.

An Interview with Peter Fisher by Cric Johnson (2012):

If there were such a thing as homeopathic royalty, Peter Fisher would easily fit the bill. And that's not just because he is physician to Her Majesty Queen Elizabeth II, as well as both Clinical and Research Director of the Royal London Hospital for Integrated Medicine–the largest public sector

provider of holistic medicine in Europe (formerly called the Royal London Homoeopathic Hospital).

Of at least equal importance is that for the past 25 years he has served as editor-in-chief of the journal Homeopathy, the only MEDLINE-indexed homeopathic journal. MEDLINE is the medical research database of the US National Library of Medicine at the National Institutes of Health and is considered the gold standard of published medical research. In his role as editor of the journal and author of numerous published studies, Peter brings to homeopathy what it so richly deserves–serious consideration, assessment, and refinement by the most rigorous methods of science.

Trained at elite Cambridge University, Peter is qualified in both homeopathy and rheumatology and is a Fellow of the Royal College of Physicians. (The Royal College is the oldest medical society in the world. Fellowship is a select honour bestowed by Royal College peers.) He is also a Fellow of the Faculty of Homeopathy (The Faculty, established in 1844 and incorporated by an act of British Parliament in 1950, regulates the education, training and practice of homeopathy by the medical profession in the UK). Peter is a member of the World Health Organization's Expert Advisory Panel on Traditional and Complementary Medicine, and he chaired the WHO's working group on homeopathy.

Can't be too bad if the Royal Family uses it.

HONEY
– see Bees and Propolis

Medicinal uses for honey
- moisturises skin when added to eggs and flour
- acts as an antibacterial and powerful antiseptic to cleanse and heal wounds and prevent scabs from sticking to bandages
- kills viruses and bacterial infections when mixed and eaten with raw, minced garlic
- boosts energy, reduces fatigue, stimulates mental alertness, strengthens immunity, provides minerals, vitamins, antioxidants

- restores eyesight, relieves a sore throat, makes an effective cough syrup
- prevents heart disease by improving blood flow and prevents damage to capillaries
- regulates the bowels, cures colitis and irritable bowel syndrome (IBS)
- acts as a topical soother for burns
- reduces inflammation and pain
- promotes faster healing
- reduces anxiety and acts as a sedative, creating calm and restful sleep
- alkalises body's pH
- protects against the formation of tumours
- relieves indigestion and acid reflux
- heals peptic ulcers
- makes a great lip balm and refreshing herbal wash or lotion
- destroys bacteria causing acne and prevents scarring
- flushes parasites from liver and colon
- heals diabetic ulcers, with topical applications
- reduces bitterness when mixed with powdered herbs for topical applications or when taken internally
- smooths and exfoliates facial skin, reduces surface lines, softens dry skin on elbows and heels
- enhances athletic drinks when added to green coconut water
- relieves hangovers
- protects hair from split ends as a hair conditioner. Honey rinse promotes shiny hair
- softens hard water by adding it to bath water
- speeds metabolism to stimulate weight loss
- improves digestion with natural enzymes
- acts as an effective cleanser when mixed with lemon and warm water first thing in the morning
- cures vaginal yeast infections and athlete's foot (anti-fungal properties)
- relieves hay fever (by chewing on honeycomb)
- protects topically and internally against pathogens such as Staphylococcus aureus, pseudomonas aeruginosa and methicillin-resistant Staphylococcus aureus (MRSA)

- builds immunity to hay-fever allergens by mixing honey and bee pollen, taken early in season
- quenches thirst and relieves heat stroke
- stops hiccups
- lessens the effects of poisons and toxins
- has mild laxative properties
- relieves asthma when mixed with black pepper and ginger
- controls blood pressure when mixed with fresh garlic juice.

Honey and cinnamon

- Mixing honey, cinnamon and hot water in varying amounts relieves arthritis, bladder infections and abdominal gas, lowers low-density lipoprotein (LDL) cholesterol and improves digestion. Additionally, it kills the flu and other viruses, slows the ageing process, restores hearing and relieves bad breath.
- Applying honey, cinnamon and hot olive oil topically prevents hair loss as well as stops a toothache.

Honey as food

- Make salad dressing using honey.
- Sweeten baked goods with honey instead of sugar.
- Smear honey on toast for a mid-afternoon energy snack.
- Preserve fruit by adding honey to water and pouring over fresh fruit in canning jars.
- Make fresh fruit jams with honey instead of sugar.
- Use for making honey, wines and beer.

HOUSE CLEANING NATURALLY
– see Bicarb Soda

People may not realise that their household cleaners can be quite damaging to health. So, if you are putting your healthy food on badly cleaned surfaces, in glasses, and hand basins, etc., the food could be contaminated.

Easy and natural all-purpose cleaner

A citrus-vinegar cleaner is easy to make and will leave your house smelling clean and fragrant. All you have to do is place some citrus peels in a glass jar. Cover them with white vinegar and let the jar sit for 2 weeks. After that time has passed, remove the peels from the jar and dilute the vinegar with water in a ratio of 1:1. Pour it into a spray bottle, and use it to clean glass, windows, bathrooms and countertops. You can even mop floors with it!

Get your cutting board spic and span

Cutting boards can be a breeding ground for germs, particularly when raw meat is cut on the same board as fruits and vegetables. If you do want to clean a board, use a lemon and some salt to clean it.

First, sprinkle the cutting board with some coarse salt. Then take a lemon with the cut side down – one that has already been squeezed will work fine – and scour the surface while squeezing a little to release some lemon juice. After letting it sit for a few minutes, simply scrape the dirty liquid away. Use a clean cloth to give the surface another rinse, and you're good to go!

Some cutting boards made from Camphor Laurel trees don't need this as the wood has inbuilt protection. Though they need reoiling by flaxseed oil as it doesn't get rancid.

Clean your drain with chemical solutions

Forget the harsh drain cleaners, which are full of all manner of unpronounceable and risky ingredients. If you've got baking soda and white vinegar on hand, you have all you need to unclog your drain naturally. First, flush the drain with boiling water and then add half a cup of baking soda. Then pour in a cup of vinegar and wait for the bubbles to subside, then run some hot tap water down your drain for about a minute and you're done.

Make your carpet smell fresh

You can make a natural carpet freshener easily by combining 2 cups of baking soda with 10 to 20 drops of the essential oils of your choice. The baking soda will lift stains and deodorise, while the essential oils will disinfect and leave a pleasant aroma.

Lavender is a good choice for a springtime floral scent, while orange, lemon or lemongrass will give your room that citrusy fresh smell. You can also combine oils to create a custom scent. Sprinkle this mixture lightly on your carpet and let it sit for a few hours before vacuuming thoroughly.

HYDROGEN PEROXIDE

Commonly called Peroxide

There is not a microbe on the planet – bacterium, virus, or pathogen – which will survive a strong mixture of hydrogen peroxide.

It is the cheapest, most effective disinfectant and, once more, not used in hospitals as big pharma controls what goes into the hospitals.

Hydrogen peroxide is simply water with an extra molecule of oxygen attached to it So simple and so effective.

It is available in many strengths, but for most household uses you will generally always use the 3% solution which I am using in these comments.

I've used it since childhood to put on cuts and grazes. Love watching it bubble up white as it kills whatever is there. If it doesn't, then I know there is no infection.

Of course, like bicarb and apple cider vinegar, it can be used in so many ways apart from the often-known use for bleaching hair.

There are many simple disinfection products that could clean hospitals but cost little and therefore not used.

As a mouthwash and teeth whitener

A tablespoon of peroxide (sold over the counter) solution in a cup of water can be used as a mouthwash. Swish for up to 60 seconds once a day, but don't swallow and be sure to rinse your mouth out afterwards. This can also help whiten teeth at the same time. You can also dip your toothbrush in and brush your teeth with it and will also help to kill bacteria on the brush.

To whiten your washing

Add a cup of peroxide to your load of whites in place of harsh chemical bleach. You can also remove stains from clothing by blotting stain with peroxide and then rinse promptly with cold water to avoid bleaching the fabric. Remove yellowing from fabric by filling a sink with cold water and 2 cups of peroxide. Soak for at least an hour, rinse in cold water and air dry.

As a household cleaner

Add some peroxide to a rag to clean bench tops and cutting boards and help kill salmonella and other bacteria. Half fill a spray bottle with it and then top it up with water for use as a bathroom and toilet disinfectant and cleaner. Mix peroxide with 2 parts water in a spray bottle and use on areas affected by mould. You can try straight peroxide for areas like bathroom tiling but be careful on the strength in relation to painted items as it may bleach them.

To combat colds and flus

Fill the cap of a bottle of hydrogen peroxide with the liquid, lie down on your side, and pour it into one ear. After a few seconds, the liquid will bubble. Lay with the peroxide fizzing for 5 or 10 minutes and then shake the peroxide out. Repeat on the other ear. You should experience results within 12–14 hours.

To clear up pimples and blackheads

Wipe your face over with it, and after repeating the process for a couple of days the blackheads have start to disappear. To help clear up pimples and blackheads, use a clean cotton ball to generously dab hydrogen peroxide onto skin. Do this twice a day, every day.

To grow better houseplants

Mix up an ounce (30 ml) of hydrogen peroxide into a cup of water and spray the solution on to your houseplants. This will help them to grow greener and more lush.

To oxygenate your body

Rub peroxide onto your skin to deliver oxygen through your pores and into your system. This is a great way to speed up detoxification and promote the elimination of toxins through your skin. You can also add 2 cups of 3% hydrogen peroxide to your bathwater for a detoxifying bath.

As part of cancer therapy

Cancer cells thrive in an environment that is deprived of oxygen. So, to help eradicate signs of cancer, it is important to alkalise and oxygenate your blood. Find an integrative or naturopath doctor who you trust and has experience administering ozone.

I

INSECTS

I find spraying colloidal silver over bites (including wasps) clears the sting almost immediately.

Also, putting something oily on before going into areas you know you could be bitten also helps, as they can't get through oil to bite.

Tea-tree oil applied to the skin can be helpful to avoid the bites or to use after being bitten.

Mosquitos are attracted to strong-smelling odours from alcohol and the human body. Some say this is why men often seem to be bitten more than women. They are also attracted to darkness so, to help avoid mosquitos, wear light-coloured clothing which people tend to do anyway in the tropics.

Mosquitos don't fly very high, which is why you don't get them in high-rise areas and apartments. They also are not in breezy areas.

You can also make a natural insect spray with a combination of citronella, lemongrass oil and peppermint oil, which is a dynamite blend of natural plant extracts.

There are many herbs and other natural agents that are soothing to the skin after being bitten and have anti-inflammatory properties, such as aloe vera, calendula, chamomile, neem oil, lemon and lime (not outdoors as affected by the sun).

IODINE

The thyroid gland synthesises thyroid hormones, and iodine is an essential trace mineral that is crucial for the thyroid to function properly. Eating foods rich in iodine ensures the thyroid can manage metabolism, detoxification, growth and development.

Iodine is known to help against atomic radiation. There was a big rush on it on the west coast of the US and no doubt in Japan after the Fukushima explosion in Japan.

The best foods are sea plants from the ocean. I have used kelp sprinkled on my soups, salads and general food.

Other foods are cranberries, organic yoghurt, organic navy beans organic strawberries, Himalayan crystal salt and any of the sea salts such as Celtic salt and potatoes with the skin on.

There are iodine supplements, both nasal and internal, available. Your local health-food shop will give you advice on this. I have a spray which I use on a casual basis just to top up but lately haven't really checked to see if I need more.

IRIDOLOGY

– see Eyes

This is all about reading the colours and marks on the iris of the eye. A good reader can tell you your whole health history and where you are presently.

A friend of mine had been having bleeding from the vagina and had the operation that cleans out the uterus to stop it but was worried that the bleeding might come back again. If so, she might be advised to have a hysterectomy. I encouraged her to have an eye reading (Iridology). Much to our surprise, she was told it wasn't a female problem, it was the spleen which controls the blood flow in our body. She was given some herbal medicine and iron tonic for the lost blood. All OK.

Some years later with bleeding from the bowel, she had a colonoscopy and was given the "all clear". I said, "It can't be, where is the blood coming from?" So agreed to have an eye reading and was told that she had nodes all over her liver and throat, which could be cancerous or impending cancer. After 6 months of herbal and dietary treatment, she was given the all clear.

J

JOINTS

– see Cod-liver oil

One of the most proven healing and strengthening products for joints is cod-liver oil. Many people have noted how much better they are by taking it. Their joints stop clicking.

Also, for bone growth: comfrey (the old name was knit bone). You can get cream to rub into the joint.

There are also many great natural mixtures to rub in and soothe the joints. Check with the local health-food shop.

JUICE

– see Fruit and vegetables

As part of any whole-food lifestyle, juice is included. The elimination and cleansing capacity of raw juice is a great way to get in all your nutritional foods.

They are rich in vitamins, minerals and more and require little digestion as they are assimilated into the blood stream.

Juices are inclined to be alkaline, which normalises the balance of acid-alkaline in the blood stream and tissue. Over-acidity is in many conditions and dis-eases.

It also helps prevent premature ageing.

K

KIDNEYS

– see Herbs and spices

We can be stressed and filled with various toxins that need clearing out without realising the kidneys are affected.

There is a number of ways to do this, such as a bunch of parsley washed clean, cut into small pieces, put in a pot with clean water and boiled for 10 minutes. Leave to cool down, then filter it into a clean bottle and keep in the fridge to cool.

Drink one glass daily and you will notice all salt and other accumulated poison coming out of your kidneys by urination. Parsley is known as the best cleaning treatment for kidneys, and it is natural!

It is also good to use if in need of iron (for liver).

Uric acid lodges in the kidneys and is found in spinach, red meat and strawberries.

When I had kidney stones, I was I kept off those foods many years ago. I love them but keep the meat to about 3 times a week (O blood needs it) and don't have too much of the spinach and strawberries. Jugs of lemon juice in water can help cleanse.

L

LAUGHTER

Today people recognise the healing value of laughter. In fact, a doctor friend of mine said she had a patient who laughed herself out of depression. The patient got all the videos she could that were related to laughter and played them as much as possible – sometimes all day.

There are workshops for laughter, which many people love as they are great fun.

As you know, hospitals now have clowns in for children to lift their energy and relax them.

LIVER – GALLSTONES

Liver renews itself quicker than any other organ. So therefore, when treated it can have quick results in comparison to other ailments, especially cancer.

As the liver helps purify the blood and digests everything going into the body, it is of primary importance in any disease.

If you are inclined to hold your feelings in and eat foods that are uncomfortable with the liver, it will often need a detox. No need to mention what alcohol does to the liver.

Gall stones and emotional symptoms of liver toxicity can cause:

- raised liver enzymes/hepatitis
- arthritis
- high cholesterol
- autoimmune diseases – rheumatoid, etc.
- cancer – all types
- chronic-fatigue syndrome/never fully recovering from a viral infection
- skin disorders
- heart disease
- waking between 1–3 am
- heart burn/gastric reflux

- persistent hot flushes/sweats that go for more than 2 years – menopause
- premenstrual syndrome
- nausea, fuzzy head, particularly in the mornings
- gynaecological disorders – endometriosis, etc.
- headaches – migraines – particularly affecting eyes and forehead
- eye disorders
- depression/bipolar disorder.

Other problems are rage, anger, aggressive personality, resentment, bitterness, boredom, mood swings, impatience, frustration, irritability, being judgemental, talking loudly, boasting, egocentricity, excessiveness, over-striving and not being able to speak the truth in the moment. These are all shown up in symptoms for diseases.

Some doctors get people to go on a cleanse before they will prescribe medicines, etc. as they know they won't be absorbed with a poor gut and liver function.

Be honest and have a good look at the symptoms above, and you may just decide to do something about it.

LOW FAT

– see Fat, Diet, Cholesterol

There are new guidelines on statins which are given to millions of healthy people in case of heart disease and cholesterol problems. I think this is a real problem as these drugs have side effects worse than the potential of having these problems.

The mantra that saturated fat is bad for you and must be removed to reduce the risks has been drummed into public consciousness for many years. However, today many are realising this is not necessarily true.

M

MAGNESIUM

Fast facts about magnesium:

- Magnesium keeps the parathyroid gland working normally. This is the gland that controls calcium levels, which in turn is essential for healthy and strong bones.
- Aside from ensuring bone health, magnesium helps the body in other ways. This mineral also helps the body convert food into energy, reduce muscle tension and lessen the pain connected to migraines and headaches.
- Women have a lot to gain from taking magnesium. The noted benefits for women include relief from the symptoms of PMS and menopause and minimised risk of premature labour.
- Green leafy vegetables, whole grains, fish and nuts are notable dietary sources of magnesium.
- Too much magnesium can be just as dangerous as too little of it. Taking high doses of magnesium can lead to serious stomach problems. People suffering from kidney problems are also cautioned against ingesting too much magnesium.

Magnesium can be taken internally and on the skin. Many things used on the skin or under the tongue go straight to the tissues, avoiding any strain on the liver, this is easy and convenient.

It is now on doctors' check lists, whereas in the past it was mostly naturopaths being concerned with lack of it.

Magnesium deficiency is often misdiagnosed because it does not show up in blood tests – only 1% of the body's magnesium is stored in the blood. It is now known that many people lack magnesium.

It can prevent migraines, lower heart-disease mortality, manage diabetes, lower risk of colon cancer, build strong bones along with vitamin D, and more.

Symptoms of magnesium deficiency include constipation and other digestive problems, low energy, irregularities in menstrual flow, reproductive health problems and migraine headaches.

Magnesium also relaxes the body from tightness, tension, tics, spasms, cramps and stiffness. And it helps prevent the build-up of plaque on your teeth, in your heart and arteries, and even in your brain.

I have a standby container of Dr Schussler magnesium-phosphate pills, and they prove wonders when chewed for cramp.

Supplements are also widely available. They come in many forms, including oxide, citrate, carbonate, aspartate, and lactate. Suggest you confirm which is best for you.

MAPLE SYRUP
– see Cancer

Maple syrup is a natural sweetener used throughout the world. Naturally it is best to have organic when using it to help kill cancer cells. It is a food with zero known toxicity (consumed in reasonable quantities).

Studies have found that the maple-syrup samples that were the darkest were most effective at inhibiting cancer cell.

There is a recipe for daily use with bicarb in my Cancer section. Have to say I now use it at times when I would have once used honey, like on porridge.

MEASLES
– see Heart

I had measles at 2 so badly that I was hospitalised. After, from being a perfectly normal healthy child I came out with a heart murmur and turned-in left eye. I have mentioned in my **Forward** how I came to be healed.

However, over recent years several healers or psychic readers have said that at that time I got a virus that stayed in my body, lowered my immune system and undermined my health, causing many of the irritation types of health, itches, skin problems, mucus and so on that I tend to get. I've noticed that when in a loving situation or romance these symptoms seem to disappear.

Also, I think a vaccine on its own, the way it was given to my children, was okay. I think the vaccines were purer, with less chemicals in them as they are today. It has also been noticed that love can often cause various diseases to fade away.

MEAT

It has been proved that processed meats in products like salami are very bad for you due to the chemicals which can cause diseases like cancer. Obviously when they were made on the farm with fresh products, they were okay but not today as they are manufactured with several chemical poisons.

I would suggest you stop buying and eating all processed meat products such as bacon, sausages, hotdogs, sandwich meat, packaged ham, pepperoni, salami and virtually all red meat used in frozen, prepared meals. Keep it to a minimum.

Like many not-so-good things for us, processed meat products are okay now and then. I love my bacon and eggs on a Sunday, which I look forward to. Cheese, tomato and pepperoni/salami on a bread stick occasionally takes me back to my travels in Europe in my 20s.

You can protect yourself and your family from the dangers of processed meats by following a few simple rules:

1. Always read ingredient labels.
2. Don't buy anything made with sodium nitrite or mono-sodium glutamate.
3. If possible, avoid meat served at schools, hospitals, hotels or other institutions.

It seems strange that, in the past, Europe has relied on this type of meat and now it seems so bad for you. Of course, originally it was made of fresh natural food.

As I am an O-positive blood group, which is the oldest group and that of the hunter gatherer, meat is important. Even a vegetarian naturopath who I knew gave up on the "no meat" when she found there was a big difference in her husband's energy once he went back to meat.

However, meat itself is acidic, so it is important not to eat too much, certainly not more than once a day, it is more easily digested by having it done the Asian way, slivered or chopped up. Have lots of vegetables with meat at least 3 times a week.

As meat is from mostly animals that have been given all sorts of food to eat along with hormones, much of the goodness has gone and it is toxic to eat. I used to eat calf's liver (so good for iron) quite often with herbs or with chill but now only buy organic, which can be hard to find. Luckily I have an organic butcher nearby.

MELANOMA

– see Cancer

MELATONIN

When people can't sleep, one of the things they check is their melatonin. Sometimes this proves to be the problem.

It's a hormone naturally produced by the pineal gland (and the digestive mucosal cell. It is to help control circadian rhythm so we are in line with the natural light and dark cycles of the sun.

People working shift hours and/or have little sleep are most affected by it. This is even true with people living in extreme latitudes. Erratic months of day and night.

Melatonin also has antioxidant and anti-inflammatory properties, which are always helpful in preventing other health problems.

Many foods naturally contain melatonin, with some of the highest being pistachios, red and black rice, orange bell peppers, walnuts, cherries, lentils, and even coffee (though this is best to avoid in the evening).

Supplementing with melatonin may not be right for everyone so check with your doctor or natural therapist.

MICROWAVE
– see EMF, Wi-fi

Many health-conscious consumers rarely, if ever, microwave their food anymore but when they do they probably do not realise that they're not just destroying the nutritional value of the food, but the "nuke" is negatively impacting their hearts.

Electromagnetic radiation dates back to radar used during the Second World War. It was designed to create death. These waves are generated by a magnetron function that enabled airborne radar to be used during the Second World War.

Don't keep anything beside or on top of the oven as it is also affected by the radiation. It is very dangerous to cook meat in.

Microwave ovens can cause unexplained headaches, nervousness, anxiety, dizziness, vertigo, impaired cognition, depression, nausea after eating, vision problems, toothache or extreme and constant thirst. These are the genotoxic effects of damaging your tissues and interfering with normal heart and brain activity.

From war experiments, the Russians banned the ovens when they figured out how dangerous they were, but not the USA! The FDA approves nearly everything that makes Americans sick, because big pharma is there to "rescue" us with expensive drugs.

When it first came out in Australia, I heard on radio about someone who tested the water from the microwave oven.

They set up approximately 6 pot plants and watered them every day with various types of water. Only one was treated with the water from the microwave. They all sprouted except the one watered by microwaved water.

I have since heard this from other sources, which means I have never used one.

MILK
– see Cancer, Osteoporosis

"Why women in China do not get breast cancer"? **Your life in Your Hands**, is a fascinating book written by Jane Plant.

She had lost one breast and was having the usual treatments but felt she was facing death. This gave her a desire to do more research on the causes.

Her husband, a scientist, had come back from China and during a discussion about the trip it seemed there was little breast cancer or prostate cancer in China.

They started to investigate this and found there was no diary food in natural, authentic Chinese food. So, they set about changing their own food and regular diet.

If you think about it, most people living in the traditional ways in Asia, Africa and South America, and other native people, rarely use diary and cancer is not so common. That is true also of osteoporosis. Their natural foods and exercise are healthy.

MOBILE – EMF. Wi-fi
5G to rival the NBN

Recently I read that a woman in Melbourne who found a 5G antenna installed in front of her house, in the street, was very upset because within a few days she was shocked to see dead bees and flowers in her beautiful old garden, which has now more or less died.

The authorities want to be able to beam through walls for information, FAST. If it goes through walls, it can go right through us and anything in nature. The world is addicted to FAST.

Researchers and physicians have warned since the '60s about the very serious physical reactions, including acute, sudden-onset health reactions, following radiofrequency radiation (RFR) exposure.

This includes skin reactions – sunburn-like areas, burning, itching, tingling, or painful sensations, bruises, skin breaks, bleeding or oozing dermatitis, migraines and headaches, stabbing pains, heart problems such as rapid heart rate and arrythmia, fainting, disorientation or even functional amnesia, dizziness, insomnia and sleep disturbances, difficulty breathing, chest pressure, hearing clicking, ringing or buzzing noises.

These reactions can occur upon first exposure or after repeated exposures. Children may be most vulnerable to these reactions.

Front page recently was about people in a high rise suffering from all sorts of problems since the 5G was installed and were going to have to move out.

Firefighters in California have reported symptoms, and after moving away from the 5G tower their health improved.

People who have been working for many years in Silicon Valley have left due to the effects they didn't realise came from their workplace.

Like the current generation of cell phone (mobile) technology, 5G has not been adequately tested to determine its impact on health. Especially how it affects all of nature including whales.

The permits and research to allow towers are 20 years old, and where once councils could ban towers in certain places, they will no longer be allowed to with 5G.

The written advice on smartphones says to not put the phone closer than 1 inch (2.5 cm) to your head. Nearly no-one follows this, including me. The 5G towers will be hard to avoid as they will be much closer together.

Too bad about the thousands of people who can't go to their work or homes, are suicidal, can't sleep, headaches, irritable, stressed, cognitive ability destroyed, ringing in ears, fatigue, and brain fog. Many of us probably feel like this to some degree and don't know what it is.

Industry is starting to make safer products though and moving to fibre optics instead, making smart meters that are read twice a day instead of all day, improving headsets and homes.

Other sources say there will virtually be no place to avoid the radiation once LED street lights with tiny antennae attached are installed. Total coverage. It comes through the ground. When there were large towers, there were areas one could move away from.

What about on planes? Just because wi-fi on planes may comply with outmoded Federal Communications Commission (FCC) standards does not make it safe for humans.

What about the growing number of people who suffer from the electromagnetic

MOLES

Moles are quite common on some people and others don't have any. I don't know much about them but had one cut off where my hair met my shoulder as I often hit it with a comb, and it would bleed sometimes.

We all keep track of them to avoid cancer. I have regularly put some of my honey-pollen ointment (Bright's natural bees wax) on some small lumps and they have disappeared. It does the same for small skin cancers. I use it for almost anything, like sores, scars and itches. I haven't tried it on moles but could be good.

MOLASSES – Cancer

This is full of minerals and one teaspoon a day gives you all the minerals you need. Added with bicarb soda, it can help heal cancer.

MULPIPLE SLEROSIS (MS)

This affects more women than men. Look to the emotional causes. One of my healers (ex nurse) went to China to see about curing herself. She spent some years there studying all kinds of medicine and healing. She has been fine for 40 years or more since her diagnosis. Definitely worth trying natural remedies on.

MUSHROOMS

– see Fungi

There are 3 different medical mushrooms which Chinese people use, and probably more –

rishi-mushroom benefits: the mushroom of immortality

maitake-mushroom benefits: the dancing mushroom

Agaricus Blazei Murill: Tokyo's cancer secret.

<u>It is important to note that drug companies cannot patent mushrooms and other natural products.</u> They want our DNA so they can own us.

You can take them raw, powdered, liquid and infused.

A close friend, who had been learning naturopathy, used one (don't remember which), found great success in slowing a virulent cancer with a healthy diet and acupuncture for a year. He had been a huge smoker which of course she cut out. Only recently come together (I introduced them) and they were able to enjoy life to a point and resolve past relationships.

However, about a year later she turned up, crying her eyes out, telling me that he had been smoking in the garden. I had to say that maybe he could no longer keep all the food and no smoking (ex Italian restaurant owner) no matter how much he loved her.

When the cancer took over and he had to go to palliative care, the nurses and doctors were baffled that he didn't have any pain and didn't need drugs. Just acupuncture on a regular basis. Luckily they allowed it, which would have been unlikely in those days.

MOULD and MILDEW

– see Bicarb, Colloidal silver, Hydrogen peroxide

I had no idea until a few years ago that so many people can die of mould.

It is incredibly hard to clear in the house, and many people have had to throw out beautiful clothes and keepsakes.

Many know it is fatal but don't realise that spraying with bleach, etc. doesn't kill it, just bleaches it and the root system is still there, so it grows back in weeks.

Basic mould can be gotten rid of with a mixture of 7 parts naturally brewed vinegar and 3 parts water, applied with a microfibre cloth. If too entrenched, professional help is recommended.

Below are suggestions on the way to get rid of it or prevent it:

1. To kill on hard surfaces, fabrics and upholstery – a quarter teaspoon oil of cloves (available at pharmacies and supermarkets) mixed with one litre of water, then lightly sprayed on the mould. I'm thinking of using it much stronger and scrubbing with something rough as what I used wasn't strong enough in an area I had.
2. Kill on leather – ¼ teaspoon oil of cloves mixed with 250 ml baby oil. Apply 2 drops and wipe over leather. Peroxide could be good here too, but I haven't tried.
3. To prevent mould in cupboards – hang 6 sticks of chalk tied with a ribbon in the cupboard to absorb moisture. When they become damp, hang them outside to dry, then reuse. I would also put chalk in the corners.
4. To prevent in books – lay a line of chalk sticks behind the books to absorb the moisture.

Also, I found spraying colloidal silver on lamp-shade mildew worked. I didn't have to buy a new lampshade.

N

NAILS

– see Hands – Fingers and nails

NEEM

Neem is a tree that is native to India. It is an evergreen and used in the traditional Ayurvedic medicine. They use the leaves, seeds and the fruit are the most used, with the seeds being crushed for oil.

Both neem oil and the leaves are used for everything from pest control to personal hygiene. Great to use the oil on itchy skin, dermatitis and eczema.

I talked to a man selling the oil at a farmer's market, and he said "I wouldn't sell anything I can't use inside as well as outside the body".

NUMEROLOGY

I was fascinated to read a book back in the 70's on numerology by Dr Juno Jordan called **Numerology, The Romance in you Name,** and one of the things I picked to do was find my health/body strength.

Numerology goes from 1, with 9 being the strongest as it tends to incorporate all the other meanings.

Anyway, I could see why my husband and son seem to have such strong health and resistance to the effects of alcohol. They had 8 on the scale, very strong, and I had 3. Three is an emotional number. Hence my health relies on my emotions even more so than many other people.

This explains a lot about our characters, connection with others and helps understand our personal experiences.

It is quite complicated with using house numbers, our name and adding our birthday. When 2 numbers, add together into 1. You can be one number in birth and a different one in name. Even the first letter of our name has a strong meaning.

NON-STICK FRYPANS

Non-stick cookware and bakeware have become enormously popular because of its convenience. Foods slide right off, reducing the amount of elbow grease required to clean the pan. Ditto for stain- and water-repellent clothing, carpets and fabrics, and many other treated products that have emerged over the past 6 decades.

However, the per- and poly-fluoroalkyl substances (PFAS) used to create these surfaces are toxic and highly persistent, both in your body and in the environment.

Today, it is more commonly known that we should not use these pans if they are scratched as toxins are released and can be absorbed into our body. Of course, we don't really notice it happening.

Some think this can be affecting women in relation to infertility, organ damage, and developmental and reproductive problems. I think that masses of modern-day living combined with our own health or lack of it causes that problem.

These chemicals are used in a wide array of household products. Besides non-stick cookware and utensils, PFCs are used to create heat-resistant and non-stick coatings that we absorb on:

- soil- and water-repellent carpet and furniture treatments
- stain- and water-repellent clothing
- protective sprays for leather and shoes
- food wraps, pizza boxes and microwave-popcorn bags
- paint and cleaning products.

I have found it, like all of us would, very hard to give up the pans at least. Many cooking utensils have been improved to avoid scratching and absorbency, though not sure how much.

Using steel and stainless steel is best, though enamelled pans and pots are good too.

NUTS

Nuts are a great form of protein, along with many other vitamins and minerals.

Ideal to nibble, instead of cheese and biscuits, when having a drink, as they are healthier. If used **instead** of having a wine, you can lose weight.

I love walnuts used with celery and tahini, or with bananas on sandwiches. Almonds contain calcium.

<u>NUT CEREAL RECIPE - not strict, adapt it if you like</u>

50% almond meal	–	500 g
30% hazelnut meal	–	30 g
10% shredded coconut	–	10 g

10% pecans, walnuts, macadamia (lightly chopped) – 10 g

cinnamon (as much as you like)

pepitas (as much as you like)

dried cranberries (light sprinkle)

I have taken to adding sunflower seeds and lecithin as well, so don't worry too much about the percentage, add what you like.

Method:

Mix all the ingredients together into a large glass jar. I keep it in the freezer.

Use ¼ cup in a bowl with a small amount of almond milk or rice milk – enough to form a wet paste (too much milk will destroy consistency). Finish off with one tablespoon of coconut yoghurt and ½ a grated apple.

Can use goat yoghurt or sheep yoghurt and any other fruit/berries instead of apple.

Very filling though it appears to be a small serving.

I don't use it on its own as suggested above, I use 2 dessert spoons on top of my big fruit salad that I have most days for breakfast or lunch, with or without yoghurt on top. My granddaughter loves it.

O

O BLOOD TYPE
– see Blood

O is the most common type of blood. There are about 200 types of blood groups, which most of us aren't aware of. I got a real shock when I heard a man on radio talking about it.

O type goes back to the hunter gatherer. It is the most ancient common blood type. My naturopath was surprised that I am in this group, as I have a poor digestion of meat, so suggested I use meat slivered or in small pieces rather than a slab.

As I am an O which is why I am including this but you will have to check on the internet for yours as far as best food to eat and best to avoid. Also, don't be too strict, slowly ween yourself off things. I don't give it a thought when I'm out I just eat and enjoy whatever food is served or available. Occasionally when I feel like it, I eat some of the **no-good** ones but only small amounts

For example, coffee – only when socialising, a treat. So, this means a few times a week or none, depending on my social calendar. I think it has little effect as long as I generally follow the main range of food .

Blood Type Diet
– Type O – see Vegetables (Potato)

People with this type of blood need a high protein diet.

They tend to thrive on intense physical exercise. Tend to love their food and therefore often have a weight problem so need to be wheat and diary free. Often they have low levels of thyroid hormone and unstable functions which can cause weight gain. Though they can usually digest meat easily.

However, I don't have a good digestion and exercise is something I have to decide to do (more interesting other things to do) unless it is dancing or loving. "I could have danced all night" as the song goes.

OLIVE OIL and LEAF

Olive oil can be said to heal many things. (Sophia Loren said she uses it for everything, from face to food. I tend to do the same.)

The olive is used for oil, and the olive leaves are full of nutrients, vitamins and healing properties. Other properties include antibacterial, anti-inflammatory, anti-fungal and anti-viral.

The leaf is said to be good for fighting yeast infections, flu and virus, treating those with cardiovascular problems and lowering cholesterol. Even the twigs of the olive tree are used to clean the teeth with in Asia.

Olives must be picked before they are eaten, and they are delicious soaked with lemon and hot chilies or other combinations.

The oil is part of the Arab diet and used in many ways. Many Arabs have olive oil every morning for breakfast with humus, yoghurt and dips. It is not only delicious, but extremely healthy.

Olive trees can last for thousands of years, which I find fascinating. Usually these are in Greece or Italy.

Natural health remedies

The oil is also a treatment for hemorrhoids, leprosy, pleurisy, skin diseases, dandruff, eczema, psoriasis, alopecia and fungal infections including ringworm, and it increases sexual desire.

Olive oil is great for the complexion. I use it at least once a week on my face and neck. Often all over after a shower and not in a hurry to go anywhere, which allows it to soak in.

When it is mixed with salt, the mixture can be used as a remedy for gum and teeth problems and combed through the hair makes the hair shiny and beautiful. It is also great for anti-ageing and longevity. As we get older, we tend to dry out so a spoonful every day is helpful.

For just about any health problem you can think of, olive oil can help. Once when I cut my thumb very badly, it was bleeding like mad and I didn't know what to do. Just grabbed an egg cup using one hand and poured olive oil in. The blood couldn't get through the oil so there were a few blobs of oil and I kept my thumb in for quite some time. When I took it out, it had stopped bleeding and I was able to get a band aid.

Buying cold-pressed olive oil can become a time-consuming activity if you get serious about it. A bit like buying wine. There are numerous grades of olive oils and on the label with some companies there will be a description regarding taste and use. When you see a deep-rich green colour, it must be cold pressed. To cook with olive oil, you need to have virgin olive oil, not extra-virgin olive oil. If we get right into it, we will have several bottles for different use.

All oils should be kept in a dark, cool place and kept out of the sunlight. Olive oil remains good for 6 months after opening the bottle or can.

OSTEOPOROSIS
– see Bones, PH

"A joyful heart is good medicine, but a broken spirit dries up the bones" – from Proverbs 17:22.

Dried plums are great for bone health: also dates, figs, raisins, strawberries and apples.

A naturopath told me that acid in the bones causes the problem, so it is important to eat alkaline food. Use a pH strip to check how acidic you are. Under 5 means you are prone to any dangerous disease. Needs to be above 6 to be OK. Ideally 7–8. Coffee is only 450 so, though good for you in many other ways, best not to have too many cups and make sure it is pure, not instant.

The drugs they give people for osteoporosis can of course have side effects. Those who avoid drugs as much as possible are successful with natural methods and of course weight-bearing exercise. I'm guilty of not doing enough of that.

No-one worried about it until the '90s when the current type of testing took place. Bone is not only calcium, it is made up of much more and the tests tend to show up the absorbency of the CAT scan. Too much calcium can cause blockages in the body.

OXYGEN

There are now centres sometimes attached to hospitals where oxygen is used to heal all kinds of problems.

When oxygen is used as a treatment, it improves the blood vessels, which can then help prevent or heal tumours thus increasing.

Oxygen can heal, and it can kill, so it is perfect for infections of all types. **The only safe way to use oxygen at high enough levels to kill all cancer cells is when it is used with carbon dioxide.**

We can fight cancer with many tumour-reducing substances, but without oxygen as the primal substance in abundance our efforts won't work.

I find cutting off the oxygen to warts is successful. When a band aid is kept on the wart, cutting the air all round, it drops off in about 6 weeks.

 Many people don't use natural remedies because it can take time and patience so they naturally take the quick way of surgery and drugs. Though often it is only the symptom being treated rather than the cause. Therefore, it can come back at some later stage, maybe in a different place.

P

PARASITES

My friend's mother was very ill. For about a year, she couldn't leave the house, was always throwing up and runny tummy. The doctors even put her in hospital and did a restart of her heart. Nothing was working.

My friend heard me talking about a natural therapist who was able to help me with a mystery problem, so she and her sister thought "I'll try anything", even though both were nurses and unaware of other forms of healing.

Her mother was diagnosed by the naturopath with parasites and allergy to oats. They had been giving her oat porridge every morning to give her strength.

She was up and running before long and enjoyed a long-distance ride within a month or two to see her granddaughter's wedding in the country.

Symptoms of intestinal parasites

Some of the most common symptoms and signs of intestinal parasites include:

- digestive problems including unexplained constipation, diarrhoea, or persistent gas
- skin problems including unexplained rashes, eczema, or hives
- muscle and joint pain
- fatigue
- lack of satisfaction after meals
- constant hunger
- teeth grinding during sleep
- anxiety
- itchy skin
- yeast infections
- loss of appetite
- iron deficiency
- itching of the anus or vagina.

The most common parasites are tapeworms, roundworms, flatworms, hookworms, and whipworms.

Pinworms, whipworms and hookworms are all types of roundworms that can cause digestive problems, mood swings, abdominal pain, brain fog, and weight loss.

Hookworms, in particular they can work their way outside the gut lining to feed on your blood, leading to anaemia.

Parasites are known to kill about 70% of animals. Many people aren't aware they have them. Kissing your animals is not a good idea, even though most pets get regular de-worming they also have other diseases that get passed on.

Parasites are also in raw meat and vegetables and slowly weaken your immune system, causing all sorts of health problems that seem to be hard to cure. So, it is also ad-vised we take worm tablets about every 6 months, maybe a couple of times as they lay eggs that don't get killed in the first round.

Natural way of clearing parasites

Cut off a large leaf of Aloe, wash and cut into about 2 cm piece and then place in a glass of water and cover. In a few hours or next morning, drink it before anything else.

It will kill parasites and clean the bowel. It tastes bitter, as many such plants do.

I believe there is some kind of an electronic rod waved over the gut with a frequency that does the trick but I have not seen or used it. Have to say I'm lazy on this and just get the pills from the chemist.

PARKINSON'S DISEASE
– see Coconut

Gluten has been shown to extend into the nervous system. So going on a gluten-free diet has shown that it diminishes the symptoms.

Also, I would use the neurological integration system (NIS) healing that my acupuncture/Chinese medicine man uses. it could possibly improve the situation.

PH

– see Hydrogen peroxide

PH is a rating of acid in the system.

As you probably know, fish tanks have to be tested for pH in the water for the fish to survive. If it is important for fish, it must be important for people. Especially as we are 70% water.

You can get pH ribbons at the health-food shops. The more acidic you become, the more likely you are to go down with a severe illness. Best to be at least 6. Anything below, you are likely to be vulnerable to illness. To test, I put some spittle in an egg cup then test. Some use it on their urine.

You can check the water you drink with it and other liquids. If the testing is too acidic, nearly yellow, (greener the better) it means that your acidity will block out the good things you are eating or any health products.

Usually, if the water is too acidic it is a good idea to get a water filter as it is blocking/absorbing our medicines and nourishing food, be they natural or from the doctor.

I notice some use their filtered water for drinking and forget about the fact they need to use it for cooking, ice blocks and so on.

PHONES

– see EMF – Mobile – Wi-fi – 5G

It is common for people to wake round 3 – I do – and find it difficult to get back to sleep. This can have a lot to do with all the electronic gadgets we have, including the smart meters and laptops which all emit radiation. Also, towers to feed these items send out microwave radiation with high frequency. It will be worse with 5G. In Chinese medicine, 1–3 is the liver and it moves into lungs, 4–6.

One of the biggest problems in today's time is getting enough sleep. More and more documentaries and articles are written about the problem.

People are having to use sleeping pills, which is not good for their health.

A concentrated effort needs to be made to clear many of these devices from being anywhere near you at night. At least a metre away. Best to do it an hour before turning off the lights. Turn them off and unplug as they still radiate from the main switch.

I have found checking the wall behind your bed for radiation is important and can be very hard to do anything about if living in a flat and can't move the bed in some rooms. You can buy meters for testing. My friend had to move her bed when I tested and later changed her bedroom to avoid the radiation coming through the wall. Her sound-system radiation in the other room was coming through the wall

PLASTIC

Check whenever you buy bottled water.

Most of us buy bottles of water without any idea what kind of plastic is being used to make them. Chances are most of us have never even been told what to look for (I certainly hadn't).

Luckily, every plastic bottle indicates what it's made of, and with a little know-how, you can learn what to look out for so that you can avoid certain chemicals. Also used for recycling.

Leaving a plastic bottle in the car and the heat exaggerates the toxin. Here's what all the symbols mean:

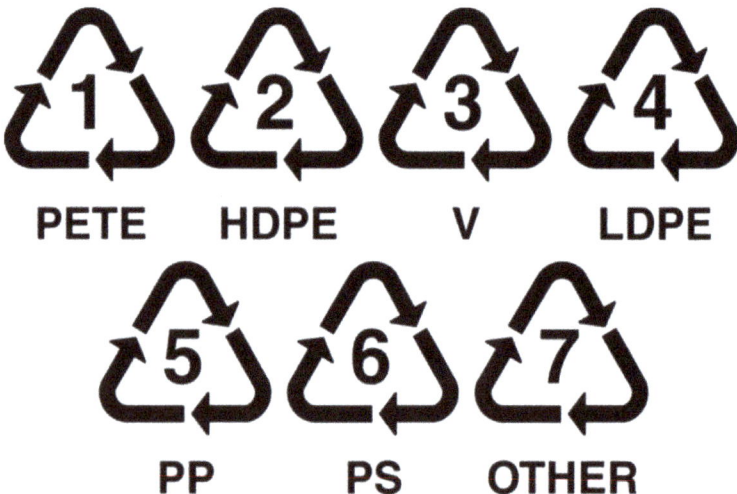

PETE   HDPE   V   LDPE

PP   PS   OTHER

PET/PETE

Polyethylene terephthalate, commonly referred to as PET (or PETE), is the most used type of plastic and is used for most drink bottles that are intended for single use only.

HDPE/HDP

High-density polyethylene (HDPE) plastic, sometimes referred to as HDP, is the stiffer plastic used in milk-gallon jugs, detergent bottles, and some toys and plastic bags. HDP can be relatively safe.

PVC/3V

Polyvinyl chloride (PVC) is a flexible plastic used to make food wrapping, teething rings, toys for pets and children, and bottles of cooking oil.

LDPE

Low density polyethylene (LDPE) releases no chemicals into water, and it is not used in the production of water bottles. It is, however, used to package food.

PP

Polypropylene (PP) is a white or semi-transparent plastic that is often used to pack yoghurt and syrups. It's tough and lightweight and doesn't melt when heated, which makes it relatively safe.

PS

Polystyrene (PS) is a cheap, lightweight plastic that can be used in a manner of ways. It's usually found in disposable styrofoam drinking cups, egg cartons, takeout containers, and plastic utensils. Not good for reusing.

PC/Unlabelled

Polycarbonate (PC) is likely the most dangerous category of plastics as it was designed as a sort of catch-all for other uncategorised plastics. These plastics can leach a lot of chemicals into food and beverages and should be avoided whenever possible.

Plastics such as bisphenol A (BPA) are shown to interfere with the productive system along with several other diseases as it is also mixed into the aluminium lining in drink cans.

Now we also know that plastic never really breaks down. It becomes tiny flakes and is now found almost everywhere in the world and therefor consumed by us and the animals and fish we eat. This can eventually cause health problems and death.

STOP using it where possible. Use glass for storage instead of plastic containers. We have liked plastic because it is so light and easy to throw around.

At least some packaging and containers are now being made from natural products and more recycled products.

PORRIDGE

– see NUTS

Porridge is a great way to start the day giving you a range of protein and vitamins. I don't eat it every day as I like variety of breakfasts Not so keen in summer either.

The recipe below can be rearranged to add sunflower seed and other ingredients. As I don't use oats due to my O-blood diet, I leave them out. I have halved this recipe as it is too much for me. I soak the ingredients for a while before I eat it. Cook it until slightly runny (to avoid milk) and serve with maple syrup,

½ cup oats

½ cup rolled quinoa

1 tablespoon amaranth

2 tablespoons goji

Can add ¼ tablespoon of chia seed.

Also, can add chopped, cranberry, fig, date, or other dried fruit. I put it in the bowl and pour porridge on it to soften it.

PROBIOTICS

Probiotics are used to help digest food. Various tablets that help this are found in the shops and they are not all in the refrigerator, which I find is a problem though no doubt best as it is live.

A teaspoon of apple cider vinegar in a glass of water is good to sip at meals as it helps digestion and swallowing my pills.

Also, many fermented foods such as tofu, kimchi and sauerkraut are excellent probiotics and are good for all areas or health.

PROSTATE
– see Cancer – Milk – Pomegranate

When it comes to benign prostatic hyperplasia (BPH), the herb saw palmetto berry has been found by many to be better than the drugs from the pharmacy.

Q

QUINCE

– delicious made into a paste to have with our biscuits and cheese. It is not a fruit which is commonly eaten. Though used to be cooked the same as apple (stew).

QUINOA

– from South America is used for salads and porridge instead of rice and has become very popular.

QUINSEY

– is hardly known but still happens. It can cause the throat to become so swollen you can't breathe.

Strangely my neighbour's son was getting married years ago and ended up with quinsy about a week or two before the wedding. He could hardly breathe and was taken to hospital.

I thought it was because he hadn't talked or cleared anger about the behaviour of his future bride in previous weeks. She was staying out late at night with girlfriends and be-having like a single woman (marriage was over in a very short time).

R

RADIATION
– see EMF - Wifi - Wireless – Mobiles or Cell phones

Not only do the heads of children absorb more radiation than those of adults but previous assessments of their exposure have not taken relevant factors into account.

When seen in a colour test of the brain, it is frightening to see how far the radiation gets in.

So much education today is on computer screens and on laptops, which attract radiation to the area of the body the laptop is on. I was amazed to read about a young man getting cancer in his legs where his laptop sat. His legs often felt burning hot. This is not surprising as the number of antennae can be about 5 on the computer or mobile.

Overuse has created addiction and schools are beginning to ban them in class because they distract the children from concentrating on what is being taught.

Today it is of great concern as it is dumbing down children as well as bad for their health, ability to resolve their own problems and social behaviour. Most no longer read book and magazines. They can't concentrate for very long even on many old movies.

Bluetooth

When this came out, I remember reading a lot about how bad the radiation was for us but that is never mentioned now. However, little official research has been done on it and we are exposed to it full time in our cars. Often, when I get in the car, I feel a bit weak and dizzy (at one stage it was always passing a certain roadside building area) which was scary. I wonder if it is the Bluetooth but brush it off as I can feel like that at other times.

In 2016, tests done on Antarctic krill found that navigation was disrupted by exceptionally weak radiofrequency fields. Research showing insect cell-death from 6 minutes of weak wireless exposure was added to previous similar findings on Bluetooth.

REIKI 1 and 11

I learned **Reiki I** (hands on) and **Reiki II** (distant healing) in the '80s from Beth Grey, who was taught by the lady who Dr Usui, (the inventor) had trained in Japan before the war. He had spent many years searching for how to heal the way Jesus did. He sent her to USA (Hawaii) before the Second World War broke out. After the war, she went to California.

It has been such a help for me with aches and pains, wind, sprains and stress.

Once when I had sprained my ankle at the bottom of a Blue Mountains walk, I managed to keep going as not too bad, but after sitting down to coffee at the top found I couldn't walk. All the way home I did Reiki on my ankle and for some time once home. The next day people were ringing to see how I was and were amazed that I was fine except for a slight pain.

Beth told us once that one of her clients had been amazed that he had felt the Reiki she was doing 8 floors above with someone else. It flows through you and out, so there is no fear of catching something with your hands on from some-one else. I know it is working as my hands begin to get hot and, if taken off before cooling the other person or myself, get that feeling you get when a hot water bottle is lifted off.

Another time a friend had grabbed a hot oven dish, which she was inclined to do, and had several scars to prove it. I grabbed her hands between mine and tried to pull away to put them under cold water or something else. I made her stay with me for some time until it stopped stinging.

She was very surprised to see no blister and the next morning no mark of any kind.

Most amazing to my son (and me) was that after a 4-hour operation putting plates on his wrecked foot and ankle, he was sitting in bed feeling good, no real pain. He suddenly felt so much pain and seemed to feel something moving around in his leg. He said he might have to take morphine to handle the pain. I put my hands on the leg plaster.

Once it eased off, I took my hands off. I'm sure it helped in his healing by repositioning some screws or whatever. He was so wrapped in how much better he felt afterwards that he later went around putting his hands on other people in the ward. He keeps saying he does Reiki, but hasn't done the course or been spiritually aligned. Though there is some degree of healing in the hands for everyone. We all tend to put our hands on ourselves where it is wounded.

I heard a man share at a Reiki 2 group that he had avoided a serious heart attack when travelling way out in the west due to his wife using it on him and ringing many friends to do distant healing while he was in the small hospital. Doctors were a bit surprised he didn't get worse and warned him to see a specialist once home.

Reiki can be done on the driving wheel in the car for safety and to plants in their pots which are looking very sad. In fact, as Beth used to say, "Don't waste your hands when sitting". She meant do it on yourself while watching television and any time.

REFLEXOLOGY

I love this form of healing as the results are so easy to measure and feel.

It is used on your hands and feet and is about massaging the sore places which are blockages. It can be very painful, but I know that means I have a lot of congestion there that needs to be broken up. It can take weeks to clear your feet from pain, which is a great help for our backs and health.

These sore spots are at the bottom of the spinal meridians. Acupuncture can also complement the healing.

Some use it as a soft way to relax but I want to use it for blockages. It is hard to do to yourself when it pains but easier to stand with someone else doing it.

My original reflexologist told me that he had a client who was a golfer and recently couldn't raise his arm above his shoulder, because of the pain. When he gave his client a few treatments, the golfer was able to swing his arm again.

S

SALT

Living in India in the '60s, I had regular lime-and-salt drinks, which were delicious, and ensured that we had enough salt to stop hydration. I had similar in Bali many years later.

However, I went off commercial salt in the '70s due to kidney problems and used vegetable salt for a long time. Now, there are all kinds of different natural salts such as Celtic, Murray River and Himalayan. I use those as they are full of minerals and good for my health.

Overweight people are often eating too much commercial salt (as well as sugar) and it can be one of the foods which retains fluid. When they feel hungry, they eat but often all they need is water.

Without appropriate amounts of sodium, your body may have a difficult time cooling down after intense exercise or activity. When the body is hot, you sweat. If you do not have enough sodium, your body may not sweat as much and you may then become overheated. This could result in a stroke or exhaustion as well as dehydration.

SELENIUM

Selenium is a trace mineral and an important nutrient to fight diseases like cancer and heart disease. It works best taken with vitamin E. Both are potent antioxidants that help prevent or slow down ageing and hardening of the tissues.

This trace mineral is beneficial for:

- antioxidant properties
- anti-inflammatory properties
- youthful elasticity in the tissues
- cataracts and macular degeneration
- cancer prevention
- healthy cardiovascular system
- hot flashes and other menopause problems
- viral infections, cold sores and shingles
- neutralisation of certain carcinogens

- dandruff
- lupus symptoms relief
- sperm production and male sex drive
- arthritis.

Natural sources of selenium are lobster, tuna, shrimp, oysters, fish, herring, liver, egg, ham, beef, bacon, chicken, lamb, veal, Brazil nuts, oats, brown rice, garlic, broccoli, wheat germ, whole grains, mushrooms, red grapes and sesame seeds.

SHINGLES

– is related to chickenpox

For natural healing, use:

Colloidal silver – When sprayed over the area, it stops the itching and calms the redness of the rash.

Tea-tree oil – regular applications of tea tree oil, diluted in water, dry out blistered sores. I like using tea tree on its own or with a little water if too painful. (Recently, I used it on potential cancer spots on my leg, they dried up.)

Apple cider vinegar and cayenne pepper – applied with a cloth 3 times a day and only to the areas of skin covered by the rash. Painful but not as bad as the shingles.

Another natural shingles treatment is with pineapple and mango, they are very highly alkaline. Lately, I find if I am chopping these I will get violently stinging and itchy hands. I have poor circulation there and often itchy. I just keep rubbing the fruit into my hands for as long as I can stand the pain, then run them under water. I find they are so soft and no longer itchy.

There are enzyme-rich fruit. So, start eating 3 daily portions of either pineapple or mango, both of which contain proteolytic enzymes that can strip away the protective outer layers and heads of the viruses.

Shingles can heal in a week or so using this approach. I also know that homeopaths and herbalists have had quite quick success in healing.

Hippocrates, that wise philosopher and doctor, stated many centuries ago: **"Let food be your medicine and medicine be your food".**

SLEEP

– see EMF -Radiation – Yawn -WiFi

The average person spends approximately one-third of their life sleeping, which is why it's so important to make sure your bedroom is protected from EMF (electromagnetic field) disturbances. (This is why electric blankets are not recommended unless they have heated the bed then turned off and plug pulled out).

An EMF is an invisible zone of energy that surrounds electric devices, and wiring is very unhealthy for you.

Most beds have metal frames. Unfortunately, these metal frames and metal box springs can amplify and distort the earth's natural magnetic field, which can lead to a non-restful sleep along with a range of other symptoms including:

- headaches
- hyperactivity
- nightmares
- depression and fatigue
- eyestrain

For muscle cramps – see magnesium.

Cats, ants and termites have an unusual characteristic in common: they're all attracted to geopathic stress zones.

Geopathic stress is natural radiation that rises through the earth and becomes distorted by weak electromagnetic fields, created by subterranean running water, certain mineral concentrations, fault lines and underground cavities.

I have tested lying on or putting the bed in the right place to avoid geopathic lines. Hard if there isn't somewhere else in the room to put the bed.   This is important for a good sleep and health.

This is why it's so important to avoid sleeping where your cat sleeps in your home as if it is located near a geopathic stress fault. Your cat will likely find it and sleep near it. If you don't have a cat, look for areas where plants do not thrive, ant hills are built, or termites congregate. These are all signs of a geopathic stress zone.

At least sleep in a bed next to the animal not with them.

It is fascinating to get a reading on the computer for your house. Orgone Effects company has a product called Geoclense which can be of help in lowering the energy.

An old-fashioned way is to use a diviner. They still use them for water divining. I wandered around my room with mine (they can be made from wire coat hangers). I reacted to my bed but, asking questions, it was more about me than the bed.

My sleep and lack of it

At least ½ hour before bed time, I stop all electronic activities as they are stimulating. Usually head to bed about 9.30, do the odds and ends, then read something not too stimulating like a biography. Settle to sleep about 10 to 10.30. I ten play relaxing, meditating type of music on CD player/ radio to relax and fall asleep to. Make sure that it can automatically turn off. I do plug it in, as batteries don't last long. I have a battery clock to help cut all electrical energy, which I put in the drawer once turning the light out. This stops clock watching if I wake up, which I often do at all sorts of hours. I then will turn my sound on to go back to sleep if I'm lucky.

I now use the awake-time for about 2 hours of reading time, which I don't seem to get to otherwise. Then lie down put my music on and sleep for another 1 or 2 hours.

The radio and phone are on aeroplane mode: they need to be at least 1 metre away from your head to avoid radiation.

I use some essential oils as a relaxant on my pillow such as lavender and marjoram and breathe them in. I sometimes use an oil on a tissue. If breathing is a problem, I have found peppermint oil (a relaxant) around the nostrils, on back of neck under the jaw, which is probably tense and, on the glands where the face/head meets the throat.

Sleeping on my right side means there is no pressure on the heart, plus it leaves the left nostril to breathe properly and relax, which is the female sleep side. It is a good idea to lay on your left side before getting up, as it helps drain the liver.

I don't use an electric blanket, which I mentioned earlier (some consider this is a cause of breast cancer, lying on your side with breast heating in one area)

Also, afternoon siesta (lie down before 2.30 pm) is a great pick-me-up if I haven't slept well (which is often) the night before. Even if I don't sleep, just lying down is relaxing, and any aches or pains I have at the time tend to disappear.

Some research shows that a siesta gives you extra years of life.

Take a bath with Magnesium Chloride and with bicarb soda, half and half. Also a warm shower can all help with sleep.

SMART METERS AND PHONES
– see Mobile, EMF, Wi-fi

The designer of Fukushima nukes and 23 nukes in the US that are like Fukushima are the largest manufacturer of smart meters in the world.

The problem with smart metering is that it will turn every single appliance into the equivalent of a transmitting cell phone, and this at a time when public concern about the safety of exposure to the radiofrequency radiation (RF) of wireless technologies is on the rise. It is really doing away with any privacy.

Years ago, when we had pagers before smartphones, a friend described them as "electronic handcuffs". They are definitely more than that now. He didn't live long enough to see the changes.

Children today cannot even fathom a life pre-internet – a life where school work involved visits to libraries and phone calls required you to stay in one spot, since the telephone was attached to the wall.

Kids spend an inordinate amount of time on their smartphones, communicating with friends (and possibly strangers) via text, Twitter and Facebook, and work hard to keep up their Snap streaks on Snapchat.

Even toddlers are proficient in navigating their way around a wireless tablet these days.

SOY MILK

One of my healers told me that a Korean client had tried everything for 3 months to stop her newborn child crying and not sleeping. She was doing the right thing by giving him soy milk.

To his surprise, he found the baby was allergic to soy milk as are many people. It is also high in oestrogen, which is not good for men. It was all the thing to avoid milk.

People got suckered into the "Soy is good for you" train back in the 1990s. As I was basically not a milk drinker, I used it instead and then began to read about how bad it could be so stopped.

Soy milk and SODD

It can affect the thyroid, cause allergies, reproductive problems, attention-deficit disorder (ADD) or attention-deficit hyperactivity disorder (ADHD), depression and more.

Regular consumption of soy milk can cause soy-originated disease and disorders or SODD.

Many people think it is good because Asians use soy and have done for thousands of years. Except it wasn't to drink like it is today. It was fermented for food.

Other ancestral, fermented soy foods include tempeh, miso, natto and traditionally brewed soy sauce.

The appearance of commercial soy milk in Asian stores only occurred in recent decades. It is a myth that Asians consume a large amount of soy foods even when fermented. It probably amounts to about a small spoon full a day.

SPRAINS and BRUISES
– see Potato, Herbal ointments, Reiki

There are several ointments that will help a sprain and bruises. Arnica and Calendula are 2 of them.

Also, many years ago (before seat belts) I had a small car crash against a small pole. I crashed my forehead between my eyes on the steering wheel. Once I got home nearby, I doused a cloth in liquid Arnica (we always had the tincture in the house) and kept it on as long as I could and as often as I could.

In the morning, there was only a slight yellow look and not much of a lump. What I couldn't help though was that when you are hit there you always get a black mark under the eyes. If I'd known that would happen, maybe I would have put Arnica there as well to prevent it.

I got lots of questions at work waitressing at the time regarding my black eyes.

Unfortunately, I don't think you can buy the liquid tincture now, but tablets and ointments are available.

STATINS

– see Cholesterol

The statin drugs prescribed to over 100 million people around the world have now been exposed as cellular poisons that accelerate ageing and promote muscle fatigue, diabetes, memory loss and more.

They seem to also cause memory loss, muscle pain, diabetes, cataracts, liver problems, fatigue and memory loss.

STEM CELLS

Many people have had great help from stem cells. I have had reports in the past from friends with the details of doctors who use them on the Gold Coast and in Sydney. I never kept the information and more recently have no knowledge of what is happening in that direction. Mostly it is only for a few problems so, as I understand it, people are going overseas and finding good results in Russia for MS. This is, of course very expensive.

STROKE

A doctor in Singapore said the most important thing to do with strokes is to put a needle at the end of each finger and make it bleed as soon as possible. It apparently keeps the blood circulating. Takes the pressure off. This was confirmed to me by my acupuncturist.

I bought a needle at the chemist that people would use for self-injections and have it in the dining room drawer. However, as I live alone, no one will know about it should it happen here.

Emails and flyers tell us how to check if you think someone has had a stroke. **FAST** (Face, Arms, Speech).

SUGAR

– see Diabetes

Sugar is known to be addictive. Tests on children have shown they may learn something today and forget it to-morrow. Very hard for them with regards to school work and spelling.

Doctors have put this down to sugar affecting the brain. They are recommending not to give children anything but water if they are thirsty. You can put some lemon in it which adds to the water value. This is very hard if they have been used to soft drinks but cut as much as possible until they get used to it (dentists say the same).

I know a nanny that told me the hyperactive grandchildren she looked after were eating a lot of sugar content stuff when she was babysitting for some weeks. She cut this down considerably and they were a lot less hyperactive.

People who have **constant sugar cravings** will find that it can be a result of some form of blood sugar (glucose) im-balance and not enough protein.

Often when we eat of lot of simple or high glycaemic index (GI) carbohydrates, they break down into glucose very quickly, so we feel energetic and satisfied for a short time after we eat but then have a bit of a low and "crave" sugar or carbs to lift those blood glucose levels again. Foods that do this are sweets, chocolate and white refined things like white bread, pastry, flour and white rice.

If you change your diet to include low GI carbo foods – such as unrefined brown wholegrain breads, flour from the breads, high fibre fruits, brown rice, rice crackers, and veggies, combined in each meal with good quality protein – you will find you don't crave those other foods.

SUNSCREEN

– see Plastic – Skin – Vitamins

A growing body of research clearly shows the absolute necessity of vitamin D for good health and disease prevention. However, despite vitamin D's role in keeping your body healthy, most people are likely to be deficient in the "sunshine vitamin".

Our vitamin D levels have dropped because of being scared by those spreading misinformation that the sun causes melanoma and skin cancer so people believe it. However, it is now known that we need a small amount of sun every day if possible. We need to expose our skin and do away with sunglasses for some of the time.

Recent research has also revealed yet another benefit of sun exposure beyond the protective benefits of producing vitamin D, namely the production of nitric oxide – a compound that lowers your blood pressure.

Your sunscreen may in fact not be very healthy. This is because many chemicals are being used to make it which are poisonous. You can read the labels, but if you don't know what they mean it doesn't help. The sunscreen can pose a grave threat to the ocean environment. These sunscreens are especially not safe for coral reefs.

The world's most popular reefs are at risk because of a common chemical found in all types of sunscreens: oxybenzone.

There is fresh concern that nanoparticles found in some Australian sunscreens and cosmetics may be potentially harmful to humans, wildlife and the environment.

There are several true sunscreens being made but mostly available in the health-food stores.

As I go to the beach early (helps to get parking) for a bit of sun and a swim, I use coconut oil with some jojoba oil in it and stay about an hour to hour and half, leaving by 10 to 10.30 am, to catch vitamin D. Late afternoon is also good as sun can be dangerous between 10–3 though the vitamin D is activated then.

SUPERBUGS

Superbugs have developed by mutating in response to the drugs that would normally work. We could be back dying from cuts and infections that we have found a cure for. We are immune to the current treatment. One of my grandfathers died of septicaemia when he was 42. That would not happen today. I also had it once.

The World Health Organization calls superbugs an increasingly serious threat to global public health, while a report commissioned by the United Kingdom warns that superbugs are becoming completely resistant and could result in 10 million deaths a year by 2050.

In recent times, though, they have found that 2 simple non-toxic and inexpensive vitamins have the potential to wipe out drug-resistant bacteria and reverse diseases that result from them. Big pharma is not interested as it wouldn't be able to get much money out of it. These vitamins are vitamin C and vitamin B3, given in high doses.

During Covid 19, I saw a video of a man who was on his last legs in hospital in a bad way and one of the doctors or a friend insisted they try a massive dose of vitamin C. Massive doses are not available for the general public. He left the hospital a day or so later feeling fine. Never heard mention of it on television again.

SWINE FLU

– SPANISH FLU – see Homeopathy, Vegetables/onion, Vaccination

Homeopathy can provide quick and inexpensive relief for symptoms of the flu. A system of medicine based on the principles of "like cures like", homeopathy uses plant, mineral and animal sources for natural flu remedies. It is based on ideas from Egyptian medicine. Modern use dates back to the 1800s.

In the 1918 flu in the US epidemic, the mortality rate of people treated with traditional medicine and drugs was

30%, and those treated by homeopathic physicians had mortality rate of 1.05%.

Gelsemium (homeopathic) was practically the only remedy used by many people. No aspirin and no vaccines.

They used homeopathy to treat Spanish flu in the US Navy on a troop ship during the First World War there had been 81 cases of flu on the way over to Europe. The report was "All recovered and landed". Every man received homeopathic treatment.

As the virus was not isolated until 1933, many believe that the epidemic was a vaccine reaction.

In another situation, there was a typhoid outbreak that doctors tried to suppress. They used a stronger vaccine, and it caused a worse form of typhoid, paratyphoid. But when they concocted an even stronger vaccine to suppress that one, they created an even worse disease, Spanish flu.

Good food, clean living, rest and exercise are the best way to avoid flu and Covid 19. Most of the people I know do this, and if they do get the flu or Covid 19 it is very mild and creates a natural immunity. Others go every year for the flu shot and still get it as has happened with Covid 19.

Other nutrients that have been shown to enhance the immune system, such as echinacea, vitamins C, D and E and beta-carotene, zinc, and elderberries are recommended.

T

TEA

There are a great variety of teas. Possibly it has many other uses but, like coffee, there is a mass of information on it. I'm sure you have developed your own taste in teas. Japanese, Sri Lankan and many Chinese teas are the basic ones.

However, there are also shelves full of herbal teas in the health-food shops, which are good for all sorts of health problems.

Herbal teas are best without milk or honey to get the real flavour. I like all teas weak, though herbal teas need time to be absorbed by the water and black with no sugar. However, many use honey instead of sugar. The water also needs to be below boiling point. As I don't use milk, I put a little cold water in so I can drink it straightaway.

TEA-TREE OIL

Treatment of cancer with tea-tree oil has been shown to slow the growth of tumours and lesions already in action. Plus, it helps boost the body's immune system to help combat the cancer at an even higher level.

Using tea tree oil to help cure skin cancer could mean the end of painful, disfiguring surgery to remove cancerous tissue. Stops my little skin cancers which might normally be burned off. Took me months to heal after one was burned off.

This versatile oil is used to treat conditions like psoriasis, herpes, respiratory problems, warts, sunburns, in addition to other bacterial and fungal skin ailments. Also, it helps clear up acne and cold sores which I use it for.

I have used it on fungus under and on top of my toe nails and it cleared up. For years I tried all sorts of other herbal creams and powders.

I have used it as a pest spray in water for about 30 years.

TEETH

– see Bicarb – Dental

Teeth are related to the meridians so if a certain tooth is playing up it could be the actual organ in the body that is inflamed or vice versa. Some people with long-term health problems have found that when they had their teeth or mercury fillings removed, their health has improved.

THYROID

– see Iodine

Thyroid deficiencies are extremely common due to lack of it in our food, while we also ingest toxins like chlorine and fluoride in our water, pest spray and poor food.

In Japan, there is more iodine in kelp seaweed and similar items of food.

I know many women take drugs for thyroid but it can be improved with better foods like kelp and seafoods. It seems to give more health problems to women than men.

There are also varying natural remedies for thyroid which are successful. I use a supplement.

TICKS

– see Colloidal silver – Parasites

If you have problems with pets where you live, get a spray bottle and add 1 cup of water followed by 2 cups of distilled white vinegar. Ticks hate the smell and taste of vinegar and will easily be repelled by this ingredient alone.

Then add 2 spoons of almond oil, which contains sulphur (another natural tick repellent). This makes a repellent that will also deter fleas and other pests I would think. Mix in a few spoons of lemon juice, citrus oil or peppermint oil (not good for animals that lick their fur), and this will repel ticks and fleas while also creating a nicely scented repellent.

Spray onto the pet's dry coat, naturally avoiding sensitive areas including eyes, nose, mouth and genitals. If you are outdoors for an extended time, take some with you to spray on 2 to 3 times per day.

For the family, use a spray bottle and mix 2 cups of distilled white vinegar and 1 cup of water. So that it smells nice, add 20 drops of your favourite essential oil. Eucalyptus oil is a calm, soothing scent that also works as a tick repellent, while peppermint and citrus oils give off a strong crisp scent that also repel ticks.

After mixing the solution, spray onto clothing, skin, and hair before going outdoors. Reapply every 4 hours to keep ticks at bay and examine your skin and hair when back inside to make sure no ticks are on the body.

There are many suggestions as to how to get rid of ticks. Another is to apply a glob of liquid soap to a cotton ball. Cover the tick with the soap-soaked cotton ball and swab it for 15–20 seconds, the tick will come out on its own and be stuck to the cotton ball when you lift it away.

Many years ago, my naturopath suggested regular rubbing of garlic into the paws of animals, which can prevent fleas and ticks from attaching themselves to the animals. Most bugs of any kind hate it.

u

ULCERS
– see Colloidal silver – Baking soda

I didn't realise that older people are very slow healers, and when I had a sore on my lower leg, which didn't heal with my previously helpful potions, I went to the skin doctor. He told me I had an ulcer and cleaned it up, added some ointment and a silver dressing with a compression bandage. I went back for dressing every 2–3 days, and it was cleared in just over a week. I'm mentioning this because I was fascinated that he was using silver, which was different from the past.

While checking out some Band-Aids, I discovered there are some now which have silver in them. Obviously, the medical profession is remembering how successful the use of silver was in the early part of the 20th century.

I know if I'd gone to a herbalist or naturopath, I would have been fixed. I just went to see the doctor as I had pre-cancers removed by him with local anaesthetic and was given a skin graft so followed through with the ulcer.

My acupuncturist says the slow-healing red lump after the sore is treated is due to lack of circulation, so he needles me there for a few sessions and it clears up.

V

VACCINATION
– see Homeopathy, Swine Flu

There was no natural immunity to our diseases in countries like Africa, America, Pacific Islands, etc. before they were taken over by Europeans. Hence there were masses wiped out. It also happened in the reverse, which most of us are unaware of.

Got a bit surprised when I heard a doctor on the radio say that syphilis was brought to Europe by the Indians. It wasn't clear to me which Indians as they were talking about something else, but I just assumed it was the American Indians. Doesn't really matter, it just shows that people around the world had different diseases to contend with. It had been unknown in Europe before.

In the past a lot of diseases and illnesses were passed on quickly due to poor hygiene and lack of knowledge as to what caused it. Once we developed better hygiene and found out about the causes of some infections, they virtually died out in those areas but continued in the less-aware areas.

Vaccinated v. unvaccinated is the question

This is something that millions of people want to follow or are forced to follow the government insisting on all kinds of vaccines as they believe in it though don't know what's in it. Others don't want their children to have vaccinations due to previous experience and research which shows there is mercury and aluminium in the vaccines.

This includes masses of doctors who have found good reason to avoid vaccines or want to do it when they think it is right for the child, or want to apply a different amount, but are forced to apply it as ordered.

In the USA, 5 year olds can have up to 19 vaccines in a month. That can't be good for anyone, let alone a child. That is a vast number of chemicals for the body to integrate.

Recently, many parents are now rebelling in the US: apart from not wanting the Covid 19 vaccine, they don't want any vaccines.

In recent years, they have found in the USA numbers of health problems that are much worse than in other countries. Could that be due to vaccinations?

Vaccine schedules are much lower in Europe and here. I, like many, would say that as a child grows the last thing you want is to have various chemicals added to their body.

Before the regular shots came in for our children, a few children would get very ill with one of these diseases as I did with measles (talked about at the beginning of the book). Strangely, as over time my 2 sisters and brother got the usual diseases, I didn't.

Though, I got German measles at 16 when I was at work (no-one else did) and in London looking after the children – I got mumps from one of them (the others didn't) and their mum did too.

However, they felt fine and had to look after me in bed as I was very ill for a week or more. Their father went away for the time as he didn't want to get it as it can cause sterility in men, which I didn't know before. One of the guys I knew also got it very badly from where? I wondered now and then, was he sterile. We were in our 20s.

This just says to me we are all different and what works for one doesn't for another, and there are many obstacles in life to overcome in one form or another. Nothing is perfect.

The basic triple antigen given to my children in the 60's seemed to have been okay as I can't recall hearing of side effects from friends or anyone else, but in later times the contents of the vaccines became, from what I've read, more toxic.

I remember reading in a Sydney paper about 4 years ago a heading and article about a breakout of whooping cough in the western suburbs. The children who had been vaccinated had caught it but not the unvaccinated. Later I wished I'd cut it out and kept it. This was a few years before the Covid 19.

This is a list of what can now be in a vaccine (March 2013) – not the Covid 19 ones. They are quite different :

- aluminium hydroxide
- aluminium hydroxide/phosphate
- aluminium phosphate
- borax
- egg protein
- formaldehyde
- gelatine
- gentamicin (antibiotic)
- kanamycin (antibiotic)
- monosodium glutamate (msg)
- neomycin (antibiotic)
- phenol
- phenoxyethanol
- polymyxin (antibiotic)
- thiomersal (mercury compound)
- yeast.

The aluminium and mercury are the main concerns regarding vaccines. A certain amount is considered safe. However, that is for one item but add that to all the other products with them in it makes a lot of mercury and aluminium.

It has now been proved that people with dementia and similar problems have aluminium in the brain and people are now advised to use stainless steel for cooking rather than aluminium pots and pans to help prevent these problems.

Many studies in the past have shown that unvaccinated children are generally healthier than vaccinated. Some people who are vaccinated have ended up with the disease again many years later.

It is simply a case of whether vaccines are really as safe and effective as they are marketed.

Thousands of people have been asking that question regarding Covid 19 vaccines due to masses of people who have chosen or were forced to take them and are now very damaged – or dead? How can a vaccine be safe after a short time of testing. (Usually there has to be years of testing) and no results reported? How good is it if you had a bad reaction to the first one and must have a booster? That is not a vaccine. How can so many people who have been vaccinated get sick with Covid 19? Vaccine in the old days, so to speak, was to last for many years or life.

ALL VACCINES SHOULD BE BY CHOICE.

Vaccine clearing
- see Pineapple

A close friend of mine received this from a well-known healer:

- vitamin c 500 mg – 4 times a day
- lipoic acid 600 mg – 1 tablet 3 times a day
- greens 3 times a day.

The healer knows she also takes Protandim every day (one of his products).

He said to begin one week before the vaccine, not after she had the vaccine.

She didn't ask him how long to continue afterwards. The main thing is to help get rid of the heavy metals.

Also, all over the world it is suggested to take zinc, vitamin D and C as a basic start for healing and immunity.

I think there would be several other things that would be helpful so suggest you check with a naturopath, herbalist, homeopath or holistic doctor.

VARICOSE VEINS

Varicose veins are swollen or enlarged veins that occur mostly in the legs and thighs in ageing or obese women, as well as in adults who stand up for long periods of time.

They tend to be surface veins rather than deep veins, so they are seldom a health risk, but they can ache. However, they don't look good and many people want them cleared which today can be done without much trouble. Check with the doctor.

My mother took the naturopath's advice for her varicose veins. She used a big, old kerosene can previously used for honey and now very clean with the top cut off. She couldn't find something deeper to reach her knee.

Most days she put it in the bath filled with water and sat on the edge of the bath with her legs in there and read for 20 minutes. As it didn't quite reach the knee, you could see the mark that showed the difference in the veins where the water ended. They had lost all the lumpy look and not so obvious. She had quite a few.

Also, when I was pregnant, I was told by the doctor to sit when ironing and whenever watching television to have my legs up on a table or footstool to take pressure off my legs. I still do that and have had next to no problem with varicose veins.

VEGETABLES
– see Juice, O diet

I have not put in all the vegetables available, just those that I have used or know about. They may inspire you to check the internet for others.

Blending is superior to juicing

A juicer extracts the juice of fruits and vegetables but discards the pulp into the waste chamber of the extractor. The pulp often contains the most curative parts. On the other hand, blending liquefies the whole fruit or vegetable and keeps the fibre in the blend instead of discarding it.

High-powered blenders can break down the cell walls of fruits and vegetables, which releases all the nutrients that the body can readily absorb.

Personally, I don't like mixing vegetable and fruit much. They sometimes seem to be contradictory. I like tropical fruits with each other. Melons with each other, berries with stone fruit and so on.

Originally, my naturopath way back said melons should only be eaten together because of their effect on cleansing. Also, they said some fruits and vegetables have a bad effect if put together. I notice the blenders throw a lot of different stuff into their recipes. Especially banana with a lot for the nice creamy taste. However, it can cause mucus in some people.

Recently it has been found eating just one serving of leafy green vegetables a day takes a decade off an ageing brain. Must admit I don't juice as much as I'd like.

Asparagus

It can be a good detox. Even the tinned product does just as well. Have to say I am not that interested in it but I am using it a bit more than I did.

Asparagus has been found to be very helpful with cancer. If you puree it from the tin and take 4 tablespoons in the morning and 4 tablespoons later in the day over a month, your count goes down considerably.

Bamboo

Abundant in Asia though now easy to get here, bamboo can be used in so many ways: supporting hair, nails, and building collagen, rejuvenating skin and joints, framing houses, creating furniture and fabric.

The shoots are used in Asian cooking and have been discovered as helpful in healing many diseases and health issues. Obviously taken in various forms which you can explore.

Bamboo was recorded as being consumed by the Chinese during the Ming Dynasty (AD 1368–1644) and found in a note from the Tang Dynasty (AD 618–907). It is literally one of the most useful plants on the planet. Amazingly it is the tallest member of the grass family.

Beetroot

Anything we can eat that bleeds as red, and as readily as the beet, deserves our immediate respect as it nourishes our blood and circulatory system.

The beetroot also is great for blood pressure as it dilates the blood vessels. And in ancient times it was legendary in its ability to enhance virility and act as an aphrodisiac. Now we know more about it, it makes perfect scientific sense.

Very tasty grated in salads and the juice can be mixed with celery and carrot. Also, the leaves are used in salads.

Broccoli

Broccoli is another vegetable that helps prevent and treat cancer especially combined with the sprouts and eaten at least 3 times a week. However, it needs to be raw to get real value (like most fruit and vegetables), used in salads and juice.

A quick stir-fry would still have some value. Better to have some than none.

Celery

Celery is rich in vitamin A, vitamin C, B complex vitamins, folic acid and vitamin K – as well as the minerals calcium, copper, iron, zinc and potassium. It also contains potent antioxidants.

Great in juice combined with other vegetables like carrot. I love it on a sandwich with walnuts, using tahini instead of butter. Very popular at a party as finger food, the hollow filled with cream cheese, cut into pieces, sprinkled with a little salt and pepper.

Cucumber

Cucumber is full of vitamins B1–3, vitamin B5, vitamin B6, folic acid, vitamin C, calcium, iron, magnesium, phosphorus, potassium and zinc.

It is very refreshing, so great with spicy foods and very tasty with yoghurt (goat or sheep). Having slices on your closed eyes is relaxing. A piece rubbed over a mirror in the bathroom will stop the fogging. Eat a few slices before bed to avoid a hangover. A slice well rubbed over anything that needs cleaning will give a shining finish, such as the tap or a pair of shoes that need polishing.

For the garden you can put slices in an aluminium pie container or similar and it will do away with grubs and bugs in the garden. They hate the smell of the combination.

Onions

Onions when cut and left for a time in a salad or sealed in the fridge can be poisonous, which would surprise everyone. They are a huge magnet for bacteria.

Most of us blame the mayonnaise (not home made) dressing if anyone gets sick from a potato salad, but it is the sliced onion causing it.

In the past I have used a half a cut onion which has been left in the fridge. Now, I have changed to buying small ones used for pickling along with large ones for cooking.

Onions and health

In 1919 when the flu killed about 40 million people in the world there was a doctor in the USA who visited farmers to see if he could help them combat the flu.

Many of the farmers and their families had contracted the flu and died. The doctor came upon one farm and to his surprise everyone was very healthy.

When the doctor asked what the farmer was doing that was different, the wife replied that she had placed an unpeeled cut onion in a dish in the rooms of the home, (probably only 2 rooms back then). The doctor couldn't believe it and asked if he could have one of the onions. He placed it under the microscope and found the flu virus in it. Obviously absorbed the bacteria, therefore, keeping the family healthy.

Of recent time, some people have reported that no-one in their office or hair salon had got sick with flu as they left cut onion in bowls around or on the desk.

Potato

When I was first pregnant, I put on weight and near the end the doctor said if I continued, I would have to go in to hospital. In those days we were only allowed to put on a certain amount of weight. I didn't think I was too heavy.

Anyway, I thought, "What makes you fat?" All I could come up with was potato and salt (retaining the fluid). Most people didn't have weight problems in those days. So, I stopped potatoes and salt. Used Veggie salt from the health-food shop.

When my son was born, I weighed less than when I started my pregnancy. Amazing. Didn't have to worry about it when I had my daughter.

Of course, I did eat potato after I had my son. However, about 20 years ago I started to slowly work on using the O-blood diet and it says potatoes are not to be eaten (I use sweet potato at home and don't worry about when I'm out). This helped me think that this way of eating is right for me.

Potato cure for bruising and inflammation:

My mother broke a bone in her knee while she was away, and being Sunday no doctor around in those days. So, she made a poultice of shredded potato and strapped it on. When she finally saw the doctor, he was amazed there was no swelling.

Since then, I have used the poultice on a sprained ankle which was so bad that I had to have something in bed to stop the weight of the covers on my ankle. Got up the next day right as rain.

Once a friend called in after he had been kicked in the upper leg and was limping around in great pain and worried that he wouldn't be able to work the next day at the flower markets.

I sent him home with a grater and a potato. The next day he had no trouble going to work.

To make a poultice, grate a potato and use a piece of cloth to put it on, then bandage it into place. Put some plastic or Gladwrap over that and then something warm as it can get cold and wet. When you take it all off, you will notice that the potato has gone black and smelly.

Good for haemorrhoids. Take a slice of potato and cut a hole in the middle to fit the haemorrhoids, then sit on it. Use some firm pants or tape it on to hold it in place if you move around, but it takes the inflammation and pain away.

Pumpkin

A book on the Japanese camps in Thailand said that the only thing that was fresh and growing secretly was a pumpkin plant. They ate all of it when the pumpkin appeared. Found they were surprisingly well after the war, which the author put down to pumpkin.

When I went to the UK early '60s, a lady I worked for as a mother's help said pumpkin was only used to feed the cattle. People didn't eat it. One day she gave me a surprise when I arrived home from my day off. She had prepared pumpkin chips, thinking this was the way we ate them. Great idea isn't it? We now get sweet potato chips, maybe pumpkin is next.

Due to the above situation and for many more reasons, Australians eat them. At home we always had to eat the skin because, as is the case in most products, it is often the most healthy part.

Sweet potatoes
– see Vaccine

Sweet potatoes are loaded with vitamins, fibre and appealing flavour.

As it comes in several colours, the darker the colour, the higher its nutrient content. They also contain high amounts of potassium, calcium, vitamin C and are rich in many other cancer-fighting compounds

Sweet potatoes contain an astonishing 600+ carotenoid compounds to help fight and prevent cancer. Along with vitamin A, sweet potato is a powerful antioxidant and helps to protect against DNA damage in cells that could otherwise set the stage for cancer.

It is now used for making sweet pies, chips as well as baked. If baked or mashed, sprinkle it with cinnamon and nutmeg with a little butter. Delicious.

VIRUS
– see Vaccination

We all have lots of viruses in our bodies and some have had infections. Most of us are unaware of how to protect ourselves from the problem.

Viruses are very tiny germs, much smaller than bacteria. They are made up of genetic material with a protein exterior. They have some unique characteristics.

There is a long list of diseases caused by viruses, including:

- some colds
- influenza
- chickenpox
- hiv
- lymes
- some pneumonia
- shingles
- rubella
- measles
- hepatitis
- herpes
- polio
- ebola
- small pox
- mumps
- epstein barr.

They are very difficult to treat with conventional medical approaches.

Vaccinations for the flu, measles, whooping cough and Covid 19 have not been shown to be consistently effective.

However, there are several natural approaches.

Fruits and vegetables can also become infected with viruses, which surprised me. Canadian folk have combined cranberry juice and citrus extract in a spray for shelf produce such as lettuce, strawberries, etc. This spray turned out to be very effective for virus prevention. Most other sprays used are for the bacteria.

Preventing and treating viral disease naturally is possible due to scientific evidence that a handful of vitamins, minerals and herbs have been shown to be effective in prevention and treatments of many viral-influenced illnesses. Especially vitamin C, D and zinc.

VITAMINS

Vitamin A

Dancing with my dentist one night (how often do you get to dance with the dentist?) he noticed my cracked and split fingers, which I get more often when it is dry and cold. He said, "You need vitamin A". Sure enough, I found taking the vitamin A healed my hands. I have to say I took a lot more pills than recommended.

It is very good for the skin and I have been taking it again (along with a few other things such as zinc) as I have had some problems with the skin on my legs. Great for eyes too.

Vitamin Bs

The B vitamins are often unbalanced and need regular checking.

Vitamin B1 (called thiamine)

This vitamin has not been taken very seriously, just included with vitamin B pills. I asked about it recently at the health-food shop and it was shrugged off. However, it is a great help to relieve, nerve and chronic pain.

Vitamin B3
– see Superbugs

Vitamin B6

This vitamin is in many foods. Though extra may need to be taken when symptoms indicate.

It is very helpful for brain development in children, immune system, autoimmune system, inflamed bowel, alcohol dependency and more.

Vitamin B12
– see Iron, Liver

Many people are deficient in B12 – vegetarians, vegans and the elderly in particular. This means your metabolism can be inefficient in burning fat, generating energy, and absorbing vital nutrients.

Without adequate blood levels of B12, you can experience symptoms related to low energy, mental fatigue, mood changes, sleep difficulties and even occasional indigestion.

Vitamin B12 is a nutrient your body cannot do without for efficient, healthy metabolism of fats and carbohydrates.

The 2 main causes of vitamin B12 deficiency are inadequate dietary intake and the inability of your body to absorb the vitamin from food.

Vitamin B12 is present primarily in animal-food sources, which is one of the reasons we are advised against being strict vegetarian or vegan. This deficiency can result in less-than-optimal nervous system function, a tendency towards nervousness and even less-than-optimal eye health.

Vitamin C
– see Vaccine

This vitamin is a great preventer of viral infections, depending on the amount the gut absorbs.

Some organs (e.g. liver, brain, eyes, etc.) actively transport vitamin C to maintain a higher level than provided by the blood. It helps the immune system in detecting and destroying foreign microbes such as viruses that attack the nasopharynx and lungs.

Many doctors and healers use it in a high-dosage form in severe cases. Dr Linus Pauling was given the Nobel Prize for his work on vitamin C.

Vitamin D
– see Autism, Bones

It has been noted by many people that vitamin D can prevent the flu and other viruses. Also, it is used for bone development, immunity and much more.

Children and people who work in the sun (though not all day as they need protection from sun as well) are less likely to get colds, etc.

The elderly who often don't go out in the sun are now being advised to get out for at least 20 to 30 minutes to absorb it so they will be less likely to have heart attacks, the flu and soft bones. The time when the sun burns most intensely is 10 am to 3 pm, and this is also the time to absorb vitamin D. This is when to be in the sun for a very short time.

Vitamin E

Vitamin E is important to those suffering from menopause (which involves the hormones), general skin healing and much more of course. Break open a capsule and squeeze the oil on a scar, and you will find it disappearing.

Vitamin K

This is taken with vitamin D, now vitamin K activates vitamin D. I vaguely remember way, way back when I was having bleeding problems the naturopath mentioned vitamin K, which I had never heard of and haven't investigated.

W

WATER

– see Plastic, Fruit, Heart, Magnesium, Varicose veins, Burns.

Drinking water at a certain time maximises its effectiveness on the body:

> Two glasses of water after waking up helps activate internal organs.

> One glass of water 30 minutes before a meal helps digestion.

> One glass of water before taking a bath helps lower blood pressure.

> One glass of water before going to bed avoids stroke or heart attack.

Water at bed time will also help prevent night-time leg cramps. Your leg muscles are seeking hydration when they cramp and wake you up. There is also often the need for magnesium with twitching muscles and cramp.

It also enables us to digest food and improves health by supporting the organs.

I've been surprised that dehydration can be the cause of so many problems. One basic to me is nearly fainting, all dizzy at the computer while working, can cause dehydration. Now I stretch, roll my head, shrug my shoulders, get up, walk around and get a big glass of water. Add lemon juice if you don't like water or a herbal tea. Fine to go back to work.

It is also a good thing to add some Celtic salt to help absorb the water which ideally is filtered which I've had it for about 30 years. I started in Sydney when there was a lot of health problems which were said to be caused by runoffs from torrential rain into the water system.

It helps weight loss by having a glass of water rather than food.

Water v. Coke which people use to stop their thirst.

Water

Most people over 50 begin to dehydrate which causes day-time fatigue which is a slow down of metabolism. It is now suggested that 8-10 glasses of water a day can ease joint pains and can slow down hunger for overweight people.

Not enough water can trigger fuzzy short-term memory and give trouble with maths and focusing on the computer scene. It can also decrease the risk of cancer. **Water is necessary for health.**

And now for the properties of Coke:

In some areas in the USA they carry gallons of Coke in special trucks which is used to remove blood from the highway. Coke dissolves or eats through most things if left in it for long enough. Removes rust spots from cars, money left in a glass of it becomes totally polished.

Great for cleaning the toilet and removes grease from clothes. At one stage where I worked we used to suggest it (along with tomato sauce) for stains on marble bench tops. As you can see it is mainly acid.

It is so addictive to the point that many people die from the affects in a town in South America effect as it is used as a cure for everything. Even the Sharman advises it be used. There is little water in the area so they drink it all the time, but it dehydrates rather than quenches the thirsts.

Drinking water

Water needs to be room temperature as drinking it cold (especially with ice) after and during a meal can cause the oily stuff in your food to solidify and slows the digestion. Then it is like sludge in the stomach and doesn't take time to be digested, lining the intestines and therefore not getting the healthy food. This can cause cancer and other health problems.

As a child we used to have a wet cloth put on our tummy with a piece of wool (an old blanket that was cut to size for tummys and necks) wrapped around it and a big safety pin or two holding it together. We always looked away when it was happening as the cold cloth on our tummy as we didn't like it but it soon warmed up. This would bring the temperature down. It was also done round our neck to draw inflammation out.

DR MASARU EMOTO became famous for photographing water crystals. As you can from these photos. The beautiful pattern is from positive thinking and feeling and the other from nasty toxic thought.

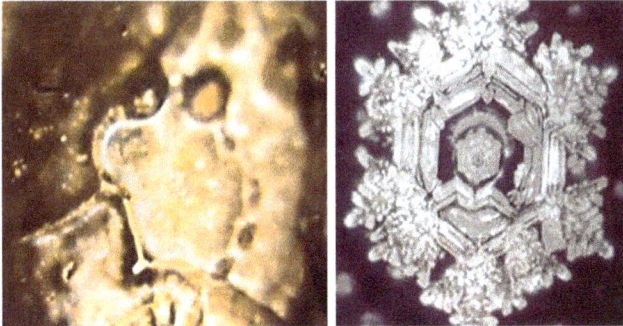

Masaru Emoto was born in Yokohama in July 1943. He is a graduate of the Yokohama Municipal University's department of humanities and sciences with a focus on international relations. In 1986, he established the International Health Machines (IHM) Corporation in Tokyo.

In October of 1992, he received certification from the Open International University as a Doctor of Alternative Medicine. Subsequently he was introduced to the concept of micro-cluster water in the US and magnetic resonance analysis technology. The quest thus began to discover the mystery of water.

He researched water all round the world and came to realise the water crystals reflect the true environment they are in, and that includes your glass of water.

In a bowl of water set on a table between 2 people, the crystals become ugly if the people behave and talk in a nasty way. When they talk and think in a loving way, the crystals became beautiful. Playing beautiful music to distilled water can also produce wonderful crystals. **Think how that must affect us, mentally, emotionally and physically, as we are largely made of water.**

Dr Emoto has written books that include pictures (above) to prove the situation, and many people think we could change our environment and waterways if we can do loving meditation. Some people are already doing this.

Maybe the great love and worship of the Ganges means that few get disease from being in the water, though the water is filthy.

Very polluted and toxic water shows hugely mal-formed crystals.

Chlorinated tap water

All over the world chlorine is added to water for public safety purposes and it does work to some degree. However, it is a chemical which we absorb into our bodies regardless of the good it does. Therefore, it can be connected to al-lergies and other problems.

Chlorine chemicals in food and pesticides are a leading cause of food allergies. If you think about the fact that we use water for all sorts of things not just drinking, we therefore absorb a lot of chemicals.

Filtering tap water is one thing we can do to avoid chorine and fluoride. You can also get filters for your shower.

One lady I spoke to who teaches swimming at the local pool said when she soaked her feet in a special cleansing foot bath (I was having one at the time) that she could smell chlorine drawing from her which is why she had the herbal footbaths often.

Currently, much of our poor health is from chemicals and electronic radiation that we are exposed to everywhere. Though there are supposedly safe levels on individual items or area when added together daily, we are in a rather toxic world and much of it is slowly spreading to those places that are being developed.

Vedic medicine says, "Drink 6 glasses or 1 ½ litres of water (filtered of course) every day and avoid diagnosed medi-cine and tablets" (saves doctor's fees). This can help pre-vent and cure disease. In other words, "Stay healthy".

Consuming water purifies the human body. It makes the colon more effective for forming new fresh blood, and the mucosal folds of the colon and intestines are activated by this method – an undisputed fact.

If the colon is cleansed several times a day, then nutrients will absorb, the action of the mucosal folds turns them into fresh blood. Water needs to be consumed on a regular basis to do the most good.

So get into the habit of drinking liquids. Liquids include water, juices, teas, coconut water, soups and water-rich fruits, such as watermelon, melon, peaches and pineapple, orange and tangerine also work.

Get people around you to remind you. Keep a glass beside you when sitting down or carry one round with you. I must admit in recent years I tend to forget.

The important thing is that every 2 hours, we need to drink some liquid.

Many people have water beside their bed to use when they wake up. **I keep a lid on my bedside water** because, as we know from Dr Emoto's work, it absorbs all thoughts and feelings, and I have some exhausting dreams that could affect the water.

Sitz bath
– see Blood

As a child, my mother used to have sitz baths (German origin and especially designed) to strengthen her reproductive area which enabled her to become pregnant with my little brother after the war.

Later, as I tended to bleeding and miscarriage, I did it too. Our naturopath had advised it. He also gave me herbal mixture and homeopathic pills.

I had to make do with a tub (I used a baby bath) of water. I filled it in the shower then sat with my legs outside the entry with slippers on and I wore something warm on top if the weather was cold. I did it for about 3 months at a time. It was a great way to catching up on my reading.

Later I read that Churchill used a sitz bath. The actual metal bath was like a chair which had a deep hollow to put the water in the sitting area.

Ordinary cold water on any area you wish to heal will bring extra circulation to the area.

WARTS

Plantar warts are very painful to start with and must be operated on, as a rule. At 16, I had to have one cut out of my heel where the hard area is joining the foot. It was a weird trip to the hospital as they put under anaesthetic. Later that day they almost carried me out to the car as I couldn't stay awake. I slept for about a day. This experience was a great help years later when it came to strength of anaesthetic.

When I was about 20, I had another plantar wart on the sole of a foot treated for weeks with acid and then had to walk back to work. This was extremely painful.

Generally, I find warts can be cleared by cutting the air supply which kills them and most things. Put a Band-Aid on to completely cut off the air. Change when needed and the wart falls off. It can take up 6 weeks.

Others have found using Bright's beeswax helpful which I buy in the health-food shop though not all have it. Rubbed in often every day.

I find this product is also good for any skin problems including small cancer like cells on the skin. When consistently used on hard areas of skin like the heel, it becomes soft. Love it on my hands. A lady that sells it at one of our markets says, "Tradies love it".

WHEAT

– see Blood type O

Modern wheat has become so genetically modified that it is now not the best food to eat.

Many years ago (before I knew about the O blood types), a friend told me she had given it up as when sprinkled to the chooks they wouldn't touch it. Glad to stop feeling bloated in the tummy. I decided then to cut back on any wheat products and it was very hard to find bread that was wheat and yeast free in those days.

Ancient man with type-O blood (oldest blood group) didn't farm and plant seeds. Hence, he ate mostly meat, seeds and fruit such as plums, dates and those older foods. No wheat or diary.

Interestingly, American foods, like corn, potatoes, avocado, tomatoes are not for people with that blood group.

Though the ancient wheats are being grown and now used for breads and pasta as they are OK. Not genetically modified.

Today, people all over the world are suffering from the effects of wheat and now are using and following a diet which is gluten (i.e. wheat) free.

WIRELESS
– see EMF, Mobile, Radiation, Wi-fi

Metals can increase wireless radiation absorption into the body. This includes phones, braces, earrings, implants, and hip replacements. Even metal implants effect the electro-magnetic radiation absorption into the body.

Usually when I go to have acupuncture, I must take off my watch and any jewellery as it interrupts the energy. Today you can buy mattress covers and other items which have magnets placed in them for healing.

WI-FI
– see EMF –Mobile, Microwave, Radiation, Wireless, Sleep

Wi-fi has an invisible but deadly effect on the world, the people and the environment.

By the time he had finished his service in the military, Barrie Trower, a British physicist, was a microwave weapons expert. He had acquired a great deal of expertise in the microwave field and he extended his research to common electronic systems, including cell phones, iPods, computer games and microwave ovens.

He was appalled to discover that microwave radiation (it was designed to kill) is ubiquitous and extremely hazardous, especially to pregnant women and young children. The risks are so great that the use of wi-fi, which is enormously popular, can lead to permanent genetic damage to your children and your children's children. Here is his personal warning in his own words:

"In the very early 1960s I trained with the government microwave warfare establishment. I looked at all aspects of microwave warfare and when I finished my time in the military, because I had a lot of expertise in the microwave field, I was asked if I would carry on with this research. We are in a new Cold War and this is why countries are developing this. And this is why all the microwave transmitters are going up everywhere because somebody, if they wanted to, could use them for other effects. The system is up and running".

Those most powerfully affected are pregnant women, children, women generally, the elderly, men and (least of all) the physically fit. Some persons appear to be invulnerable to exposure, but a significant percentage – from 47.7% to 57.7% – appear to be especially vulnerable, even though most of us might have what is regarded as low doses that represent minimal risk.

Reading this reminded me of a small group I went to about 25 years ago who were interested in energy.

One, a doctor there, had something like a Geiger counter (I now have one though maybe not as powerful) which he put near the microwave, the printer, television, etc. and all showed a danger zone. Some were worse behind than in front. This means they could eventually have a major health problem if constantly there in a small space (we were in an office).

He told us he had decided to use it at the home of a patient who was never well and always had health problems. She lived in an area of Sydney back from the harbour on a hill where there is a naval base some kilometres away.

When held up at the window facing in the direction of the base, though many houses and hills between, it registered though not too bad.

Her husband was an electrician and quite healthy. The doctor looked under the bed and found many leads backwards and forwards leading to the plugs. Once these were rearranged and **earthed,** her health really improved.

When I worked at Kings Cross at the jazz club, there would be all sorts of erratic electrical happenings now and then where I was living. Everyone would say it is probably coming from the naval base.

Many electrical items and plugs are not earthed these days. So, it is a good idea to make sure everything on your meter is earthed.

Schools around the world are removing or reducing the use of wi-fi as the behaviour and health problems have shown up since having it. Sadly, so much schooling is done now via computer.

A great book about radiation is by Donna Fisher – ***More silent fields: Cancer and the dirty electricity plague***.

WOMEN and MEN
– see Prostate - Milk

The Pill tends to deplete the body of moisture and nutrients which causes drowsiness in some women, depression and infertility, so they need to have extra nutrients.

Men over 50 have more oestrogen than women of the same age. Usually, they need progesterone, not oestrogen. Though as I understand it, oestrogen can help to stop prostate trouble.

Sadly, due to today's environment, oestrogen is causing early puberty in some girls. This means that they start their periods at 10, although they are not emotionally mature. So in their 20's they need to check for breast cancer.

High GI can influence our genes and creates a desire for bad foods.

Low GI helps decrease disease causing genes.

High amounts of carbs are common in breast cancer. Low GI: reduced stress and anxiety. Coconut flour and oil are very good to use regularly.

Prostate – needs, exercise, good food which switches the genes on for healthy living. Men need to speak up about their health and emotional problems before it is too late. I know of 2 men who ignored all the symptoms and it was too late for them to be cured.

We are now one of the fattest nations and need to change our eating and food habits. It is well known that weight is one of the causes for hip and knee replacement.

Lack of sleep causes cravings, thirst, blood pressure problems and more. Good sleep regulates them. However, it seems much of the world is having sleep problems which may have a lot to do with the electronic environment and stress.

Snacking on food can be a habit to fill in time or because we love a particular food. Hungry or not, we eat it. Alcohol problems start off the same way.

I know that when I'm feeling upset, miserable or lonely and things aren't working out, I'll get the urge (though don't follow it much) to spoil myself and have a cake and coffee/tea. If later in the day, have a wine and nibbles to soothe me in front of television. This then of course can create a habit and add weight.

I avoid having biscuits and cake in the house, so eat some nuts and dried fruit or spicey rice crackers (lots of alternatives in health shop) rather than cheese and crackers or do something else to break the habit. I keep a pack of mostly gluten-free biscuits to eat if I have a visitor pop in. Though, if at home I like one a day with an herbal tea in the afternoon.

I've found just stopping the wine and nibbles in front of television I've lost 3 kilos in a week or so. Just have nuts instead. Though it comes back as soon as I get into my old habit. Not that I think about my weight, rarely use the scales, but sometimes feel uncomfortable in the fit in my clothes which is when I go back to not nibbles etc.

I'm inclined to think that fussing over calories and scales confirms and creates weight problems. It has been proved that regular exercise (a daily walk will do) and cutting our eating too much (use a smaller plate) along with processed food and sugar is the best way of losing weight.

We need to understand ourselves and work on resolving the issues and problems we have, and we will have less craving to escape in one form or another.

X

At this stage I have no connection to anything beginning with "X".

Y

YAWN

It is so good for you to yawn, as it is to laugh.

Once when I went to a one-on-one interview, I couldn't stop yawning and worried about it as generally we think it shows boredom.

Seems that, in fact, yawning releases toxins from the liver built up from stress or poor breathing. You'll notice that people coming out of the movies will often yawn a few times because they have not been breathing properly due to excitement or stress of the movie.

I'm finding yawning is good to do when I can't get to sleep due to thinking or worrying. Yawn, yawn and it feels relaxing.

YEAST

– see Blood group, Fat, Fungus, Weight, Wheat

Yeast can be in many foods apart from those specifically cooked with it, like bread. So many people are cutting down considerably on yeast by using sough dough.

I have talked about yeast-free diets, etc. in the pages above.

There is another kind of yeast, brewer's yeast, which is good for you but I haven't investigated it. My mother used it in her smoothies.

YELLOW

– See Colours

I have been painting a large canvas of sunflowers and, in the group, people have come up and said they see happiness. Loading it into the car, a man parked nearby called out how happy he felt. That was a big surprise, but yellow is the colour of the sun and warmth. Also the most popular colour when people are asked about their favourite colour. Maybe because it is the colour of the sun.

As there is so much bad news and problems around, I suggest we all get something yellow in the house and wear yellow to lift our spirits.

YOGA and other Asian exercise

I'm sure you all have some knowledge about the varieties of yoga, which is another ancient practice, and has exercises related to the whole body. Breathing is very important for health, and this is incorporated with yoga.

Yoga is an ancient Asian practice that is spiritually inspired and is probably the first one that the world in general heard of and practised from about the late 19th century due to the European colonising. Later, as people read, travelled more, had radio and cameras, etc., **they discovered tae kwon do, zen, tai chi and so on.**

They are exercising but each move is named and based on the inner self release of energy and strengthening. It is about the emotional, physical, spiritual self which people have felt more fulfilled by, rather than just counting the number or push ups and kilometres they run.

Z

ZINC

– loss of taste

Recently I have had healing-resistant sores on my lower legs, as they were taking months to heal. My naturopath suggested I start taking 4 zinc tablets per day instead of one, and she advised me to get an ointment based on zinc and pine called Calmoseptine. This has proved to be very helpful, although I had to be patient to see results. It also helped to have acupuncture.

Zinc is one of the major minerals to take to help prevent and heal disease, clear up infections and is used in a cream to heal skin infections. We can go back to zinc instead of chemical sunscreens.

A few days after my sister died, I was on a ship which had been booked long ago, so I had to go, but all that lovely food tasted like sawdust rather than gorgeous cakes, coffee or exotic food that would cheer me up. I felt so disappointed and sad and wondered what had happened. Never heard of people losing their sense of taste except from head accidents.

Apparently, it happens after use of medical drugs and goes away in time (I wondered how long) according to the doctor. As the drugs didn't apply to me, I was mystified.

As weeks went by, I could find no answers (checked with dentist who I'd been to not so long before the trip). Eventually I checked with my naturopath and she said it was due to an imbalance of zinc and copper, and she gave me a plan on how to correct it. Luckily, copper pills were then available. I seem to have lost the information regarding how to take the 2 sets of pills. Still at least I know what it is.

Lack of zinc can cause sudden loss of hearing sometimes in one ear at a time and sometimes over about 3 days. May have ringing in the ears (tinnitus) and loss of balance (vertigo).

Zinc has been shown to be a big help in improving the hearing and therefore other health problems. Like many things as we age, we become more deficient in zinc. It is suggested that we have 30 mg a day when healthy, but when for certain situations like athletes, pregnant women and restoring hearing, 100 mg a day.

Food sources of zinc are:

- oysters, raw – organic
- calf's liver
- beef, chuck
- lamb shoulder
- unsweetened chocolate
- plain yoghurt
- cashews

I'm sure some of you would love to eat lots of oysters but unfortunately expensive.

CONCLUSION

Health, healing and happiness must come from within. Too often we think that having a new partner, a better job and so on will solve the problem. They won't. Though they may inspire you to make the changes.

Loving yourself enough to achieve the changes also develops more self-esteem. One healer will often direct you to another of the various natural remedies which can fit in with your medical treatments when needed.

It takes courage and patience (some say 28 days to change a habit) to develop new habits of eating and exercise. Never beat yourself up or feel guilty when you "aren't doing it right", as you may say. None of us can be perfect in following and doing all the good things we would like. We gradually develop what suits us. Don't waste time and money on things you don't really want to do. You may come to that at another time.

Most people in the ageing business recognise that, to really live life fully to the end,

we need to have healthy emotions and thoughts when resolving issues, removing stress and therefore relaxing more. Often then this will bring you into more personal understanding and growth and enable you to become more relaxed and happier.

Life is about 10% of what happens to you and 90% how you handle it. Learn to action situations rather than react to them. In other words assertive rather than angry.

As the saying goes, "Where the mind goes, the energy flows", so direct your thoughts to create the desire to eat better foods and experience how much better you feel after exercising, which can take many forms. Brisk walking (can be a type of mediation), dancing are my favourite exercises. Did love Zumba Gold but not so happy with venue and time so intended to take up yoga but lock down stopped that and I haven't got going with yoga.

Gradually, you will enjoy it rather than think that you **should** or you **have** to. Both are negative guilty words so far as relaxing and enjoying anything.

Aim for prevention of health problems rather than have to treat a full-blown health problem. Age is only a number. Many young people are quite old and many older people are quite young in attitudes and life style.

Good HEALTH, HEALING & HAPPINESS is all in the thinking, emotions and behaviour.

GRATITUDE and THANKS

I am so grateful to Dr Bernard Jansen (Capricorn which is my House of Health in astrology. That house is also about being of service, ie healer, pets and more) for bringing me back to life as I faded away and showing the family how to live a healthy, fulfilling life. In my 30s, I came to understand that the real source of his knowledge was developed through astrology and theosophy, as well as naturopathy, iridology, homeopathy, osteopathy and herbalism.

I am so grateful that I have family and friends whose encouragement and support, along with their conviction that the book would appeal to many people. They can't wait to have one.

I am grateful to all those teachers who added to my understanding of astrology and myself. To Beth Grey, Reiki Master, Rae Sinclair for years of personal growth. along with doctors, healers of all types who put in years of study in their field of healing. (In Germany a doctor does another 3 years in homeopathy if they wish)

Gratitude and thanks are due to many people who helped me throughout the process of bringing this book together. The book is generated from lots of notes, emails and readings, along with my reflections on them. I believe I received guidance in choosing the right people to help, through lists on the internet, magazines and referrals.

Tara's (never did get her surname) via Airtasker with her ability on the computer to put many separate notes and pages for research into one book and that includes the re formatting. it was fascinating to watch. I felt so grateful.

With much gratitude, I found my initial editor, Lisa Wood, who was a whizz with fixing my computer as well as helping me understand what editing entails. As time went by, she began a different lifestyle so it was time to look for someone to take over.

I have been very grateful to find Anne Isdale through a referral from a kind editor (not working at present) on the internet who I thought I might have been related to. She has been just right for my type of book.

I am so grateful to my friend Rod Lane, who has had the patience and creativity to bring my rough design regarding the **cover** of this book into reality.

Lastly, to my photographic award winning son Luke Feltham gratitude for the lovely **photo**.

REFERENCES

Alexander, E. (2012). *Proof of heaven: A neurosurgeon's journey into the afterlife*. Simon & Schuster.

American Psychiatric Association. (2013). *Diagnostic and statistical manual of mental disorders*, Fifth Edition (DSM-5). San Francisco: American Psychiatric Association.

Chisolm, D. (2020). *Have you got the guts to be really healthy?* Retrieved from NuFerm website: https://www.nuferm.com/product/book-have-you-got-the-guts-to-be-really-healthy/

D'Adamo, P. (2002). *Live right for your type*. Penguin Books Ltd.

De Angelis, E., de Angelis, M. (2012). *Postcards from the other side: True stories from the afterlife*. Sydney: Allen and Unwin.

Erasmus, U. (2007). *Fats that heal, fats that kill*. Summertown, Canada: Book Publishing Company.

Fisher, D. (2009). *More silent fields: Cancer and the dirty electricity plague: The missing link*. Buddina: Joshua Books.

Gawler, I. (2017). *You can conquer cancer: A new way of living*. Melbourne: Wilkinson Publishing.

Harrison, J. (1984). *Love your disease: It's keeping you healthy*. London: Angus and Robertson.

Hay, L. (1988). *Heal your body: The mental causes for physical illness and the metaphysical way to overcome them*. USA: Hay House, Inc.

Hendriks, H. (2010–2015) *Making Australia happy. Making couples happy. Making families happy*. Simon & Schuster ABC DVDs, ABC1.

Johnson, C. (2012) *An Interview with Peter Fisher*. Retrieved from World of Homeopathy website: https://

worldofhomeopathy.wordpress.com/2012/07/04/an-interview-with-peter-fisher/

Joudry, P., Joudry, R. (1999). *Sound therapy: Music to recharge your brain*. Sound Therapy Australia.

Just, A., Kall, J. (2018). *Autoimmunity and metal implants, devices, and vaccine adjuvants* (2018). World Mercury Project Partner. Retrieved from https://worldmercuryproject.org/news/autoimmunity-and-metal-implants-devices-and-vaccine-adjuvants/

King, P. (2017). *Up until now: The inspiring story of the founder of Quest for Life*. Sydney: Allen & Unwin.

Kubler-Ross, E. (1969). *On death and dying*. New York: Scribner.

Lipton, B. H. (2008). *The biology of belief: Unleashing the power of consciousness, matter & miracles*. Sydney: Hay House.

McKissock, M., McKissock, D. (1995). *Coping with grief*. Sydney: ABC Books.

Mercola, J. (2023) *Peak fitness video library*. Retrieved from Mercola Peak Fitness website: https://fitness.mercola.com/sites/fitness/videos.aspx

Moorjani, A. (2012). *Dying to be me: My journey from cancer, to near death, to true healing*. Carlsbad, California: Hay House Inc.

Plant, J. (2007). Why women in China do not get breast cancer. In *Your life in your hands*. London: Virgin Books Ltd.

Schuessler, W. H. (2023). *The simple logic of Schuessler's theory*. Retrieved from Schuessler Tissue Salts website:

https://schuesslertissuesalts.com.au/about/history/

Segal, I. (2007). *The secret language of your body: The essential guide to health and wellness*. Blue Angel Publishing.

Siegel, B. (1986). *Love, Medicine & Miracles*. Bethesda: Arrow Books.

Van der Kolk, B. (2014). *The body keeps the score: Brain, mind, and body in the healing of trauma*. UK: Penguin Books Ltd.

Zorza, R., Zorza, V. (1981). *A way to die: Living until the end*. Glasgow: Collins.

Organisations in Australia specialising in retreats, work-shops and counselling for healing cancer and other ailments, including spiritual, emotional and physical problems.

Life and Living 10-day retreat founded by Ian Gawler, who lost a leg to cancer. Yarra Valley, Victoria. 03 5967 1730.

Living Waters 10-day cleansing course and more. Kin Kin, Queensland. 1800 644 733.

Quest for Life Foundation founded by Petrea King, who was given a few months to live. Bundanoon, New South Wales. 02 4883 6599.

www.ingramcontent.com/pod-product-compliance
Lightning Source LLC
Chambersburg PA
CBHW041255040426
42334CB00028BA/3030